A FALCON GUIDE®

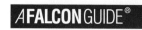

Backcountry First Aid and Extended Care

Fifth Edition

Buck Tilton, MS, WEMT

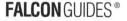

FALCON GUIDES®

GUILFORD, CONNECTICUT
HELENA, MONTANA

AN IMPRINT OF THE GLOBE PEQUOT PRESS

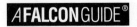
Illustrations by David Gross and Judy Newhouse

Library of Congress Cataloging-in-Publication Data

Tilton, Buck.
  Backcountry first aid and extended care / Buck Tilton. — 5th ed.
    p. cm. — (FalconGuides)
  ISBN 978-0-7627-4357-5
  1. Backpacking injuries. 2. First aid in illness and injury. 3. Wilderness
survival. I. Title. II. Title: Backcountry first aid. III. Title: First aid and
extended care.
  RC88.9.H55T55 2007
  616.02′52—dc22   2007001987

Manufactured in the United States of America
Fifth Edition/Third Printing

Contents

Foreword

Some people live or work in remote situations—ranchers, forest rangers, biologists, or guides. Many people recreate in the backcountry and enjoy nature, adventure, quiet, and companionship.

For most people a trip into the backcountry is enjoyable and healthy. We only use our first-aid kit to treat blisters and small cuts. If the unfortunate emergency arises, however, this little book offers a wealth of information, experience, and advice packed into a very small space.

Buck Tilton has been a wilderness medical educator for more than a quarter century. He distills the essentials of wilderness medicine into this simple and straightforward presentation. As you read this you will understand why so many outdoor enthusiasts are Buck Tilton fans.

This fifth edition of *Backcountry First Aid and Extended Care* is for anyone who enjoys the wild outdoors. It will give you the knowledge to handle injuries and illnesses in remote settings. It will help you get through the first minutes of a medical emergency with a structured patient assessment system. It will get you started on the right steps to properly treat and protect the patient from further harm. It will help you be a wise leader and make good decisions about when you should evacuate the patient to a physician's care.

Whether you are leading your friends, your family, your scout troop, or your summer camp, as a leader you need to make good decisions. This text reflects a mix of common sense and best practices—essential ingredients for good medical judgment.

Tod Schimelpfenig
Curriculum Director
Wilderness Medicine Institute of NOLS

Acknowledgments

This book is included in many first-aid kits manufactured by Wisconsin Pharmacal Company, and it serves as a text for wilderness first aid courses offered by the Wilderness Medicine Institute of the National Outdoor Leadership School. To the staff of "the Pharm," especially Andy Wundrock, and to the instructors of WMI, especially Catherine Stifter, much is owed by this author. But the greatest thanks go to Tod Schimelpfenig of WMI—a colleague, a friend, and one of those rare people you can always count on.

1. Introduction

Time is the essential element distinguishing first aid from extended care. When the doctor is far away—an hour or more, according to the Wilderness Medical Society—the principles of first aid are often unequal to the task of managing the injured and the ill. Consider the rough trail, the wandering length of river, or the long miles of black asphalt separating the patient from a medical facility. Think about the heat or cold, the rain, the wind, the darkness. Remember that equipment needed for treatment and evacuation may have to be improvised from what is available, and communication with the "outside world" may be limited or nonexistent. Remote locations and harsh environments may require creative treatments. All these things are the stuff of extended care.

It is the responsibility of those who play, work, and live in isolated places to be able to act appropriately in an emergency. Like all talents, first-aid and extended care skills can be learned. Excellent opportunities to gain the knowledge and practical skills were few and far between not long ago. Now they are available regularly in many communities.

Note: This book does not pretend to have all the answers. It provides principles for dealing with many serious emergencies and a few common problems. It is intended to be a reminder about what to do for those who have training and a stimulus to learn for those who are untrained. It is not intended to be a substitute for professional medical care when such care is available.

2. Action Checklist

__ Take a deep breath. *Stay calm. Take charge.* Be quick but not hasty. *Act fast—but go slow.*

__ Before stepping in, size up the situation and make sure the *scene is safe.*

__ Perform an *initial assessment*, treating the patient for any immediate threats to life or limb.

__ Perform a *focused exam and history*, examining the patient for problems and gathering information.

__ Sit down, take a deep breath, look around, and *plan what to do*. Treatment must be considered and carried out, an evacuation may need to be prepared, help may need to be requested.

__ *Stay or go, fast or slow?* If an evacuation of the patient is necessary, decide if you need to move quickly or at a more leisurely pace.

__ Keep a *written record* of the emergency. Be ready to give a verbal report.

__ *Act* in the best interest of the most people.

3. Patient Assessment System

Before you can properly care for any patient, you have to assess what is wrong with the person. An assessment is a step-by-step process. Although some of the steps may change in order, depending on the immediate status of the patient, no step should be left out.

STOP! SIZE UP THE SCENE

Take a few moments to stand apart and survey the scene, checking for specific information, before you step into the scene. These may prove to be the most valuable moments in your response to a patient.

1. Survey the scene for hazards. Is there immediate danger to you, other rescuers, bystanders, and/or the patient or patients? Make sure the scene is safe. You must do all you can to ensure you *never create a second patient*. Humans are resources who can think, help tend the patient, and participate in carrying a litter. A second patient not only doubles the trouble but also reduces the resources—the problem is more than twice as serious.

2. Determine, if possible, the mechanism of injury (MOI). Are there clues suggesting what happened to the patient, the forces involved? How far, for instance, did a patient fall, and what made up the "landing zone"?

3. Establish body substance isolation (BSI). Take proper precautions—put on rubber gloves and perhaps glasses, for instance—to protect you and the patient from germ transmission.

4. Determine the number of patients. A patient in obvious (and noisy) distress may temporarily hide the fact that you have another patient lying silently a few yards away.

5. Form a general impression of the patient. Very hurt or very sick? Not seriously hurt or only a little sick?

PERFORM AN INITIAL ASSESSMENT: ABCDE

Once safely at your patient's side, perform an initial assessment. The goal is to *identify and treat any immediate threats to life*. If you discover a threat, stop and fix it. Immediate loss of life will be from ABCDE: A) loss of an *airway;* B) inadequate or nonexistent *breathing;* C) loss of adequate *circulation* because the heart has stopped or too much of the patient's blood is leaving the circulatory system (e.g., onto the ground or spilling inside a body cavity); D) extensive *disability* from damage to the spinal cord; or E) extremes of the *environment.* At your patient's side, check ABCDE.

1. Identify yourself and your level of training, and ask for consent to provide care: "Hi, my name is ＿＿＿ and I've been trained in first aid. Can I help you?" If the patient says something like "Yes" or nods in acceptance, or even

says nothing to indicate lack of consent, you have consent to treat. (For a patient with a mental status too low to allow a response, go to the section "Airway Obstructions and CPR.")

2. Establish the patient's level of consciousness (see "Vital Signs," below), and place a hand on the patient's head to initiate spine control: "Please do not move until I know more about you. Can you tell me who you are and what happened?" The patient may identify a chief complaint: "I twisted my right knee, and it really hurts!" If the patient does not identify a chief complaint, feel free to ask what hurts.

3. Assess for A, an airway: "Can you open your mouth?" Take a look in the mouth to check for possible obstructions to the airway and, of course, remove anything blocking the airway.

4. Assess for B, breathing: "Take a deep breath, please. Good—does that feel okay?" If breathing is difficult, you need to figure out why and fix the problem (see "Airway Obstructions and CPR," "Chest Injuries," and "Medical Emergencies").

5. Assess for C, circulation: Assess for an adequate pulse (see "Vital Signs," below). There may be something you can do for a heart beating too fast or too slow (see "Shock" and "Medical Emergencies"). Then perform a quick scan for major bleeding. If you find major bleeding,

stop the blood loss. Immediately expose the wound and use direct pressure on the wound and, if possible, elevate the wound to control the bleeding (see "Wound and Wound Infection Management").

6. Assess for D, disability: Your hand is still on the patient's head. Investigate the mechanism of injury more thoroughly to decide if you need to maintain spine control (see "Spinal Injuries").

7. Assess E, the threat of the environment: Prolonged exposure to environmental extremes can cause changes in body core temperature that threaten the patient's life. The most common threat is cold. For that reason a patient should be protected from the environment—e.g., gently placed on a sleeping pad and covered as protection from cold—as soon as safely possible. This can be done now (see "Spinal Injuries") or, more often, after the patient exam (see below). The E for environment can also be an E for exposure, a reminder that you must sometimes expose parts of the patient's body to assess the extent of damage and provide immediate care, if necessary.

PERFORM A FOCUSED EXAM AND HISTORY

When the patient is free from all immediate threats to life, you need to start gathering clues. The focused exam and history continues the step-by-step examination of the patient. The goal is to find everything that is not in perfect working order.

Since these problems are not immediate threats to life, treatment can usually wait. This examination includes three phases:

Patient Exam

Check the patient from head to toe to locate any damaged parts. **Look** for wounds, swelling, or other deformities. **Ask** where it hurts and if it hurts when touched. **Feel** gently but firmly, using a massagelike action with your hands spread wide to elicit a pain response but without causing further damage. Be aware of unusual smells (e.g., alcohol) or sounds (e.g., labored breathing). If you suspect an injury may be hidden beneath clothing, you must take a look at skin level. "Go to skin to assess" is the mantra of the rescuer.

Check:

1. Head, looking for depressions in the skull, damage to the eyes, and fluid in the ears, nose, or mouth.

2. Neck, for pain or deformity.

3. Shoulders, for pain and symmetry of the shoulders.

4. Chest, for pain, ability to take a deep breath, uneven breathing movements of the chest wall, and abnormal breathing sounds.

5. Abdomen, gently pressing on all four quadrants (with the belly button as the central point) for pain.

6. Pelvis, for pain by pushing on the two pelvic crests.

7. Genitals, if and only if it seems relevant.

8. Legs, for pain and including symmetry and the ability to move the feet.

9. Arms, for pain and including symmetry and the ability to move the hands.

10. After this head-to-toe check, roll the patient found flat on her or his back to assess the back. If the patient has an injury that could have damaged the spine, the roll must be performed carefully (see "Spinal Injuries"). Press on every bone of the spine. *Note:* This is a fine time to place the patient on a pad as protection from the cold ground.

Vital Signs

Vital signs are measurements of the physiological processes necessary for normal functioning. They do not often tell you what is wrong, but they do tell you how the patient is doing. *Changes in vital signs over time are indicators of changes in the condition of your patient.* Check early, and keep checking. To better monitor a patient, record the time at which you take each set of vitals.

Vital signs include:

1. **Level of consciousness** (LOC): To check how well the brain is communicating with the outside world, use the AVPU scale:

   (A) Is the patient *alert,* able to answer questions? A+Ox4: Patient knows who, where, when, and what happened. *Note:* If the patient knows what happened, she or he usually knows the rest of the story as well.

A+Ox3: Patient cannot remember what happened but does remember who, where, and when.

A+Ox2: Patient can only relate who and where.

A+Ox1: Patient only remembers who she or he is.

(V) Does she or he respond only to *verbal* stimuli? Grimacing or rolling away, for instance, from your voice when you speak or shout? In what way does the patient respond?

(P) Does she or he respond only to *painful* stimuli, such as an aggressive knuckle rubbing into the sternum or a pinch? In what way does the patient respond?

(U) Is she or he *unresponsive?*

2. **Heart rate** (HR): Count the number of heartbeats/minute by pressing two or three fingers just above the wrist on the thumb side where you find the radial pulse. For speed, count for fifteen seconds and multiply by four. Note the rhythm and quality of the pulse. Is it regular or irregular, weak or strong? Normal heart rates are strong and regular and usually somewhere between fifty and one hundred beats per minute.

3. **Respiratory rate** (RR): Count the number of breaths/minute without telling the patient what you are doing. A patient who knows you are checking often alters the breathing rate in an attempt to be accommodating. Note also the rhythm and quality of respirations. Normal

lungs work about twelve to twenty times per minute at a regular and unlabored pace.

Note: Without a watch, you should still get a rough estimate of heart and respiratory rates. Rough guesses are better than no idea.

4. **Skin color, temperature, and moisture** (SCTM): Normal skin is pink in nonpigmented areas such as the inner surface of the lips and eyelids, warm, and apparently dry to your touch.

SAMPLE History

More information is usually gathered by subjective questioning than by objective checking. This information is known as a patient's history. Hopefully the patient will provide the answers. Sometimes witnesses are sources of important information. Speak calmly, and do not use leading questions. In other words, say "Describe your pain" instead of "Is it a sharp pain?" Be aware of your tone of voice, body language, and eye contact. Patients usually feel better and respond better if they think you are nice—but do not make promises you cannot keep. If you gain trust you must maintain trust.

The SAMPLE questions:

S for symptoms: Pain, nausea, lightheadedness, other things you cannot see.

A for allergies: Any known allergic reactions? What happens?

M for medications: Anything legal or illegal? Why? How much?

P for pertinent medical history: Anything like this happen before? Currently under a physician's care for anything?

L for last intake and output: When was food or drink last taken? How much? When were the most recent urination and defecation? Were they normal?

E for events: What led up to the accident or illness? Why did it happen?

SOAP: THE WRITTEN REPORT

In an emergency your brain tends to become a sieve instead of a bowl. The acronym SOAP reminds you to write everything down (to collect documentation) as soon as possible—as long as taking notes does not interfere with patient care. Retention of information for medical and legal reasons is important.

S for subjective/summary: A summary of who the patient is (including age and sex), what the patient complains of, and what happened to the patient.

O for objective /observations: Observations and results of patient exam, vital signs, and SAMPLE history

A for assessment: What you think is wrong.

P for plan: What you are going to do immediately for the patient and the answer to the evacuation question—stay or go, fast or slow? A part of every plan is to *monitor* the patient for changes and developing needs.

You might also add A for anticipated problems: What changes you might see in the patient.

SOAP: THE VERBAL REPORT

If you can make radio or phone contact and ask for support, you will need to give the SOAP note in verbal form. The person hearing your verbal SOAP should hear something like this:

(S) I have a 23-year-old male patient whose chief complaint is right knee pain. The patient states, "I was running and stepped in a hole and twisted my right knee."

(O) The patient was found lying on his back about 3 miles from Lander on the Middle Fork Trail. Patient exam revealed swelling of the right knee. The right knee is about twice the size of the left knee and red in color. Patient denies loss of consciousness. Patient denies pain or tenderness along the spine. There is normal circulation below the right knee. Nothing else was found.

At 3:00 P.M. the vital signs were LOC=A+Ox4; HR=78 regular and strong; RR=18 regular and unlabored; SCTM=pink, warm, and sweaty.

The patient reported the following history: No symptoms other than pain in the right knee. Patient is allergic to aspirin but denies taking aspirin. Patient denies taking any medications. Patient denies pertinent medical history. Patient describes his fluid intake as "about two quarts of water today" and his food intake as "two ham and cheese sandwiches" for lunch. He reports a clear urination "about an hour ago." Patient states he was not watching the trail closely and failed to see the hole.

(A) Based on the MOI this is not a possible spinal injury. His problem is a right knee injury that makes walking impossible.

(P) I will improvise a splint for the right knee. I am alone, and I will need a litter and assistance to carry the patient to the trailhead.

(A) I will monitor the patient for loss of circulation below the swollen knee and for loss of body heat.

4. Airway Obstructions and CPR

During the initial assessment of a patient (see "Patient Assessment System"), you may find immediate threats to life involving ABC—airway (it is blocked), breathing (there is none), and circulation (the heart is not beating). If you find one or more of these problems, you must attempt to fix the problems immediately!

AIRWAY
An airway starts at the nose and mouth and ends deep in the chest, where oxygen is exchanged for carbon dioxide. If the airway is not open all the way, it will not work.

Airway Obstruction: Conscious Patient

In a conscious patient food is the most common obstruction. If the patient can speak or cough, do nothing but watch and wait. If the patient goes silent or starts to wheeze, it is time to step in and help.

1. Confirm that the patient is choking and cannot speak.

2. Say "I am going to help" and move behind the patient.

3. Wrap your arms around him or her with one hand formed into a fist and pressed into the patient's abdomen, thumb side of fist in, just above the navel. Cup your fist with your second hand.

4. Pull in and up with a quick, forceful motion while keeping your elbows away from the patient. This maneuver is known as an abdominal thrust.

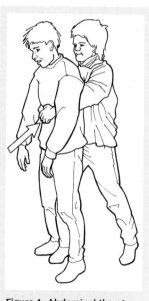

Figure 1. Abdominal thrust

5. If the object is not expelled, repeat the maneuver until it works.

Note: For patients who are very pregnant or obese, wrap your arms around the chest with your fists pressed into the sternum (breastbone) and perform the same thrusting motion. (You can perform abdominal thrusts on yourself if you find yourself alone and choking.)

Airway Obstruction: Conscious Patient Becomes Unconscious

If the patient becomes unconscious before the airway is cleared, lower her or him gently to the ground.

1. Call for assistance.

2. Open the airway with a head tilt–chin lift (see below). Look in to see if you observe an object. If you see something, get it out.

3. Place your ear near the mouth and look, listen, and feel for breathing for ten seconds.

4. If the patient is not breathing, attempt to ventilate the patient by pinching her or his nose closed, sealing your mouth over the patient's mouth, and blowing air into the patient.

5. If air goes in and the chest rises, give a second breath, and then check for a carotid pulse (see below) and other signs of circulation: breathing, coughing, and/or move-

ment. *Note:* Rescue breaths should be slow, about one second/breath, with allowance for patient exhalation between breaths.

6. If the attempt to ventilate fails, reposition the patient's head and try again.

7. If no air goes in, perform thirty chest compressions as you would do in cardiopulmonary resuscitation (CPR—see below).

8. Open the airway to see if any obstructions have become visible. If so, remove them.

9. Attempt ventilations again (see above). Keep up this sequence until the airway is cleared.

Airway Obstruction: Unconscious Patient

If you find a patient who appears unconscious:

1. Check immediately for responsiveness to a verbal followed by a painful stimulus (see "Patient Assessment System").

2. Call for assistance.

3. Open the airway. In a patient found unconscious, the most common airway obstruction is the tongue. Most airways can be opened by using the head tilt–chin lift maneuver. If, however, you suspect spinal injury (see "Spinal Injuries"), use a jaw thrust (see below) to open the airway, a maneuver that does not endanger the spine.

4. With the airway open, look for objects.

5. Look, listen, and feel for breathing for ten seconds.

6. If the patient is breathing, check for a carotid pulse (see below) and other signs of circulation.

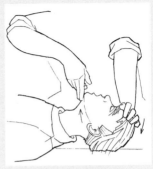

Figure 2. Head tilt–chin lift

7. If no breathing can be detected, attempt to give the patient a rescue breath.

8. If your air goes in, give a second breath and check for a carotid pulse (see below) and other signs of circulation.

9. If your air will not go in, reposition the head and try again.

10. If air still will not go in, perform thirty chest compressions as you would do in CPR (see below).

11. Attempt ventilations once again (see above). Continue this sequence until the airway is cleared.

Note: Any rescue breathing is safer in terms of your personal health and well-being if you use a pocket rescue mask.

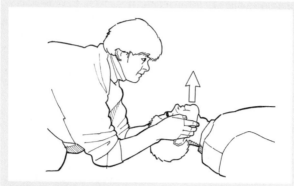

Figure 3. Jaw thrust

BREATHING

If your check for breathing reveals no respiratory activity, and your ventilations go in, and the chest rises as you blow in showing that air is getting into the lungs, that means the patient has an adequate airway but is not using it. You must keep breathing for this person.

After two initial slow breaths, however, pause for ten seconds to check for a heartbeat. A beating heart will be indicated by a pulse and/or by breathing, coughing, or movement. To check for a carotid pulse, place two or three of your fingers over the carotid artery, which is located in the valley between the windpipe and the large neck muscle, just below the angle of the jaw. If you find indications of a beating heart, continue rescue breathing by giving one breath every five to six seconds until the patient starts to breathe.

CIRCULATION

Rescue breathing, remember, is useless if the patient does not have a beating heart to push around the blood you are oxygenating with your breath. Cardiopulmonary resuscitation is discussed briefly here. According to the American Heart Association, however, CPR must be done well in order to work well: good ventilations, good compressions, minimal interruptions. CPR courses are offered regularly in most communities. Take a course, and stay in practice to do your best.

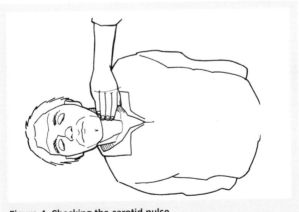

Figure 4. Checking the carotid pulse

Note: If you do not have a rescue mask and you do not wish to perform mouth-to-mouth ventilations, at least perform the chest compressions.

ADULT CPR: ONE RESCUER

1. Assess scene safety.
2. Take body substance isolation (BSI) precautions.
3. Assess responsiveness to a verbal and then painful stimulus.
4. Call for assistance.
5. Open the airway and look for objects.
6. Look, listen, and feel for breathing for ten seconds.
7. In the absence of breathing, give two slow breaths, about one second/breath.
8. Check for a carotid pulse and other signs of circulation.
9. In the absence of circulation, begin chest compressions by placing one fist on the lower half of the sternum, placing your other hand over the first, keeping your arms straight and locked, and pressing down about one-third the thickness of the patient's body. Depress the sternum thirty times at a rate of one hundred compressions/minute.
10. After every thirty compressions, give two slow breaths.
11. After five cycles of 30:2 (approximately two minutes),

check for a return of circulation. If no circulation is present, continue the cycles of thirty chest compressions to two breaths, checking periodically for a return of pulse and other signs of circulation.

Note: Any patient with adequate breathing and circulation, either before or after CPR, should be rolled into the recovery position to ensure maintenance of the airway.

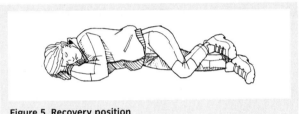

Figure 5. Recovery position

5. Spinal Injuries

Through the vertebrae (backbones) runs the all-important spinal cord. If its nerve messages are impeded by damage, the result may be permanent paralysis or death. During the initial assessment, any patient who has a mechanism for a spine injury (see below) should be kept still with calm words and hands on the head until secondary treatment can be applied (see below). *Note:* A patient found unconscious should be considered spine-injured until proven otherwise. Highly suspect mechanisms of injury include:

1. Compression/axial loading, such as falling from a height or landing on the head

2. Excessive flexion, as when the chin is forced to the chest

3. Excessive extension or rotation, such as tumbling downhill without skis releasing

4. Distraction, such as an attempted hanging

5. Penetration, as from a gunshot or stabbing

6. Sudden and violent deceleration

SIGNS AND SYMPTOMS OF SPINAL INJURY

1. Pain, tenderness, or obvious injury to the spinal column

2. Altered sensations in the extremities (e.g., numbness, tingling, unusual weakness, inability to move, and unusual hot or cold sensations)

3. Respiratory difficulty

4. Loss of bowel control

5. Signs and symptoms of shock (see "Shock")

MANAGING THE SPINE-INJURED PATIENT

If the patient's neck lies at an odd angle, it may be straightened with slow, gentle movement—performed by the rescuer—to line it up with the rest of the spine. This straightening improves the airway and makes immobilization easier. If this movement causes pain or meets resistance, stop and immobilize the patient's head as it lies.

A patient with a possible spinal injury who is found crumpled into an odd body position may be straightened with slow, gentle movement of one body part at a time. This typically makes the patient more comfortable and provides for better immobilization.

When the spine-injured patient has to be moved, say into a tent for warmth or out of an avalanche zone, move her or him via body elevation and movement (BEAM). Get as many hands under the patient as possible, with firm ones on the head. At the command of the head holder, lift the patient *as a unit* with as little spine movement as possible and carefully carry him or her to a predesignated spot. *Note:* If you have never performed a BEAM, it is best to practice first on someone who is not injured.

A patient on her or his side can be logrolled onto the back. Manual stabilization of the neck is critical during the roll. At the command of the head holder, the patient is rolled *as a unit*. A logroll can also be used to roll a patient onto her or his side in order to place a pad underneath before rolling the patient back onto the pad.

With the spine in normal alignment, the next step is to stabilize the cervical spine (neck). Ambulances carry rigid cer-

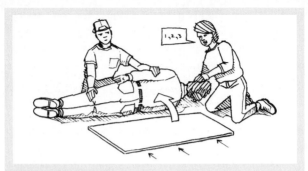

Figure 6. Logroll

vical collars. You can improvise one in the backcountry by rolling extra clothing, such as a long-sleeved fleece sweater, or by cutting off the end of a closed cell foam sleeping pad to fit the patient's neck and taping it in place.

Collars, even commercial products, do not totally stabilize the cervical spine. Hands-on attention should still be maintained, if possible, until the whole patient is stabilized in a rigid litter. In the backcountry you are often looking at a long wait for a litter, but attempting to move a spine-injured patient without one creates great risk and is *not* recommended. When a litter is available, the patient should be FOAMed in place—made Free of Any Movement—with lots of padding and straps. Avoid the voids by placing pads under the knees, in the small of the back, and anywhere there

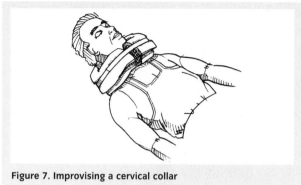

Figure 7. Improvising a cervical collar

is space that could let the patient shift. The patient's head should always be strapped down last. Proceed with care.

FOCUSED SPINE ASSESSMENT

After completing a *full* assessment on a patient with a mechanism for spinal injury, and after finding *no* signs and symptoms of spinal injury, you may choose to perform a focused spine assessment in hopes of discontinuing spinal immobilization. A focused spine assessment includes a *second* check for:

1. A fully reliable patient—a patient who is a) at least A+Ox3 on the AVPU scale, b) sober, and c) without distractions such as severely painful injuries or deep psychological distress.

2. A patient without altered sensations in the extremities.

3. A patient who denies spinal pain ("It hurts") and tenderness ("It hurts when you press on it").

EVACUATION GUIDELINES

Evacuate anyone being treated for a possible spinal injury. Evacuate *rapidly* anyone with the signs and symptoms of spinal cord injury.

6. Head Injuries

Head injuries—and here we are talking about trauma to the brain—can be loosely divided into two categories: mild and severe.

MILD HEAD INJURY

Despite the possibility of heavy bleeding from a scalp wound or the growth of a goose-egg-sized bump, serious damage is rare if the skull is intact and the brain relatively undamaged. The patient may have suffered a decrease in mental status but responded immediately to aggressive stimulation: loud shouts or forceful pinches. Symptoms may include short-term amnesia, brief blurred vision, nausea, headache, dizziness, and/or lethargy. Treat wounds appropriately: pressure from a bulky dressing on the bleeding scalp and a cold pack for the bump. Acetaminophen may be given for pain. Keep an eye on the patient for about twenty-four hours. Awaken the patient every couple of hours during the night to check for signs and symptoms of serious brain damage (see below).

SEVERE HEAD INJURY

Unconsciousness in which the patient does not respond to aggressive stimulation may indicate serious brain damage. The injury may or may not involve a skull fracture (see below). A skull fracture should always be considered severe.

Signs of a Skull Fracture

1. A depression in the skull

2. A visible fracture where the scalp has been torn away

3. Bruising around both eyes (raccoon eyes) or behind both ears (Battle's sign)

4. Cerebrospinal fluid and/or blood weeping from nose or ears

Signs and Symptoms of Brain Injury

Head-injured patients without signs of skull fracture may appear okay and then start to deteriorate. Monitor for these signs and/or symptoms:

1. Level of consciousness (LOC) deteriorates from disoriented to irritable to combative to coma.

2. Heart rate (HR) slows down and bounds.

3. Respiratory rate (RR) becomes erratic—may be fast; may be slow and labored.

4. Skin (SCTM) becomes flushed and warm, especially the face.

5. Protracted vomiting.

6. Visual disturbances that persist.

7. Ataxia (loss of coordination) and/or seizures.

8. Lethargy and/or excessive sleepiness.

9. Increasingly severe headache.

10. Pupils may become distinctly unequal.

Move the patient gently and check carefully for cervical spine damage that is sometimes associated with a severe blow to the head. Keep the patient lying down. If possible elevate the head and shoulders slightly, up to about 30 degrees. If breathing becomes excessively slow and labored, start periodic rescue breathing.

EVACUATION GUIDELINES

Evacuate anyone who does not respond initially to aggressive attempts at stimulation after a blow to the head. Evacuate *rapidly* anyone with signs and symptoms of severe head injury, especially a skull fracture and/or a decrease in mental status.

7. Shock

Shock is inadequate perfusion, a condition that results when the brain and other body cells are not getting a sufficient flow of oxygenated blood. It can occur from a great variety of injuries and illnesses, including blood loss, dehydration, a heart attack, spinal cord damage, and a severe allergic reaction. Whatever the cause, most shock patients share similar signs and symptoms.

SIGNS AND SYMPTOMS OF SHOCK

Early changes include:

1. Level of consciousness (LOC): anxious, restless, disoriented

2. Heart rate (HR): rapid and weak or thready

3. Respiratory rate (RR): rapid and shallow

4. Skin color, temperature, and moisture (SCTM): pale, cool, and clammy (but may be pink and warm with some forms of shock)

5. Symptoms: nausea (and sometimes vomiting), dizziness, thirst

Late changes include:

1. LOC: Continued decrease with eventual unresponsiveness.

2. HR: Radial pulse weakens and eventually disappears.

TREATMENT PRINCIPLES FOR SHOCK

Whatever the cause, shock can kill! Backcountry treatment for shock is limited. Early recognition and management are critical. At first *assume shock in all patients* until it is proven otherwise.

1. Treat early, before serious signs and symptoms develop.

2. If a cause can be identified, such as bleeding or dehydration, treat the cause.

3. Keep the patient calm and reassured.

4. Keep the patient lying down and protected from loss of body heat.

5. Elevate the patient's feet approximately 10 to 12 inches. (Injuries to the head or lower extremities may preclude this.)

6. Although fluids are not usually recommended, small sips of cool water may be given to prevent dehydration on a long evacuation if a) the patient tolerates fluids, and

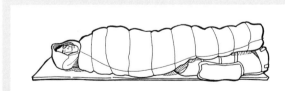

Figure 8. Shock treatment position

b) the patient's mental status allows holding and drinking from a container.

EVACUATION GUIDELINES

Evacuate any patient with signs and symptoms that do not stabilize or improve over time. Evacuate *rapidly* any patient with decreased mental status or worsening vital signs.

8. Chest Injuries

Any injury to the chest may lead to respiratory difficulty and a critical patient. A simple fractured rib (see "Fractures" under "Musculoskeletal Injuries") may not be so simple if a bone fragment punctures a lung. Air escaping the lung and collecting in the chest is called a *pneumothorax,* with its increasing difficulty breathing and a rising level of anxiety. A pneumothorax can worsen until the patient is unable to breathe adequately, a condition known as a *tension pneumothorax*, which often results in death. Suspicion of a pneumothorax calls for an immediate evacuation.

If several ribs are broken in several places, a free-floating section of chest wall, called a *flail*, often results. The flail will move in opposition to the rest of the chest wall during breathing. Flails are not common, but this condition is extremely serious. Taping a bulky dressing over the flail may allow the patient to breathe a little more easily. The tape should not be placed entirely around the patient's chest because that makes it more difficult to breathe. During the rapid evacuation—the speed of which may be all that saves the patient's life—the patient may require rescue breathing. Evacuation of the patient on his or her side, injured side down, sometimes aids breathing.

If the chest has been opened by a penetrating object, the hole may bubble and make noise when the patient breathes. This is called a *sucking chest wound,* and the hole should be immediately covered with an occlusive dressing—something that lets no air or water pass through. Clean plastic will work. Tape this dressing down with a corner left free in hopes that air collecting under tension in the chest will self-release. If collecting air does not release, a pneumothorax may develop and may progress to life-threatening tension. If severe difficulty in breathing develops, push your finger or some other object gently into the hole to release the trapped air. This treatment may be all that can save the patient. Once again, a speedy evacuation is critical.

EVACUATION GUIDELINES

Evacuate *rapidly* anyone with signs and symptoms of serious chest injury and/or anyone with increasing difficulty breathing.

9. Abdominal Injuries

Abdominal injuries may be generally classified in two categories: 1) *blunt trauma,* a closed abdominal injury caused by a forceful blow to the abdomen, and 2) *penetrating trauma,* an open abdominal injury caused by an object being forced into the abdomen. The extent of injury is often difficult to assess in the backcountry—or anywhere, for that matter. No other region of the human body has more potential to conceal serious blood loss.

SIGNS AND SYMPTOMS OF SERIOUS ABDOMINAL INJURY

1. Obviously serious abdominal injury, e.g., an impaled object or evisceration (internal organs outside the body).

2. Signs and symptoms of shock (see "Shock").

3. Blood in the vomit, feces, or urine. Blood may appear like coffee grounds in the vomit, black and tarry in the feces, and reddish in urine.

4. Pain in the abdomen persisting for more than twelve to twenty-four hours.

5. Localized abdominal pain, especially with guarding, tenderness, rigidity, palpable lumps, distention, and/or asymmetry.

MANAGEMENT OF ABDOMINAL INJURY

Generally, treat for shock (see "Shock"). Stay alert to the possibility of vomiting. Patients suffering blunt trauma should be kept in the position of comfort they choose—if no other injuries prevent this—and kept warm. If you are involved in the evacuation, comfort and warmth should be extended to patients during the carryout. In general, nothing should be given to them by mouth, but on an extended evacuation, sips of water, preferably cool, may be necessary to prevent dehydration.

The immediate seriousness of any penetrating abdominal injury, as with blunt trauma, is determined by what got damaged inside and how bad it is bleeding. With severe bleeding, shock is imminent and immediate evacuation the only chance of salvation. Over time the risk of infection may be high. General treatment of the patient is the same as for a patient suffering blunt abdominal trauma. Specific treatment will vary somewhat depending on the soft tissue involvement. External bleeding should be controlled. Wounds should be cleaned and bandaged. Impaled objects, in almost all cases, should be stabilized in place.

An evisceration, in short-term care, should be covered with sterile dressings soaked in disinfected water to prevent drying out. Check the dressings every two hours to make sure they stay moist. Cover the moist dressings with thick, dry dressings, and rapidly evacuate the patient. In long-term care (more than several hours), the exposed intestines will do better if they are flushed clean with disinfected water and "teased" back inside by gently pulling the wound open. If teasing does not work, you may have to gently push the exposed loops of intestine back inside the abdominal cavity. Then clean and bandage the wound.

EVACUATION GUIDELINES

Evacuate *rapidly* anyone with signs and symptoms of serious abdominal injury.

10. Wound and Wound Infection Management

When you are far from a doctor, three general goals will guide your management of wounds: 1) Stop serious bleeding, 2) prevent infection, and 3) promote healing.

BLEEDING

Life-threatening arterial bleeding pulses or spurts from a wound each time the patient's heart beats. Venous bleeding, which can also be serious, flows smoothly and rapidly.

A quick visual scan of the patient is often enough to detect serious bleeding—but not always! Check inside the clothing of someone wearing bulky winter gear or rain gear. Check beneath someone who is lying in sand, rocks, or any terrain that might disguise blood loss. Severe blood loss can also be internal (see "Shock").

Almost all external bleeding can be stopped with *direct pressure and elevation:* pressure from your hand directly on the wound and elevation of the wound above the patient's heart. If there is time, place a sterile dressing on the wound before applying pressure. If there is no time, grab anything absorbent to press into the wound. You can let small wounds bleed to a stop—which may actually clean them a bit.

Warning! Some wounds should not be treated with direct pressure. Pressure to a wound on a patient's neck may cut off the air supply—instead, stop the bleeding by carefully pinching the opening closed. Pressure to a head wound may push cracked bone fragments into his brain—in this case, cover the wound with a bulky dressing and press lightly but firmly.

Direct pressure and elevation may be augmented by pressing on a pressure point, which reduces blood flow to an extremity. The pressure point for an arm is the point where you feel a pulse inside the upper arm just below the armpit. The pressure point for a leg is near the groin where you feel a pulse in the crease where the leg meets the torso.

If blood loss is tremendous and death imminent, a tourniquet can be used on an arm or leg. Tie a band of material, preferably 3 to 4 inches wide, around the limb as close to the wound as possible, and snug it down until blood loss stops. Loosen the tourniquet periodically to see if clots have closed the wound. Retighten the tourniquet if you need to, but leave it in place no longer than necessary.

Note: Before touching blood or any other body fluid, it is best to put on protective gloves. If there is a chance blood may be splashed into your eyes, wear glasses, e.g., sunglasses.

WOUND CLEANING

Proper wound cleaning, closing, and dressing almost equal the prevention of infection. Cleaning also speeds healing and reduces scarring. Start by washing your own hands and putting on surgical gloves. Avoid breathing into, coughing around, or adding contamination in any way to an open wound.

Start the cleaning process by scrubbing around the wound with soap and water and rinsing the skin with disinfected water. Remove any foreign matter embedded in the wound with disinfected tweezers or by gently brushing the matter out of the wound.

The best method for cleaning the wound itself is mechanical irrigation. Irrigation involves a high-pressure stream of an acceptable solution directed into the wound, best directed from an irrigation syringe. For most wounds the best cleaning solution is plain disinfected water. For heavily contaminated wounds you can whip up a disinfecting solution by thoroughly mixing an ounce of povidone-iodine in a liter of water and waiting about five minutes. *Note:* Do not drink this solution. Draw the solution into the syringe, hold it about 2 inches above the wound and perpendicular to the wound, and push down forcefully on the plunger. Keep the wound tipped so the solution runs out. Use at least half a liter, more if the wound still looks unclean. If you don't have an irrigation syringe, you can improvise by using a biking water bottle, melting a pinhole in the center of the lid of a standard water bottle, or punching a pinhole in a clean plastic bag. If you use something other than plain water, follow irrigation with a final flush of disinfected water.

WOUND CLOSURE

After thoroughly cleaning small wounds that gape, facial wounds, or scalp wounds, you can close them with closure strips or strips of tape. Another guideline is this: If you had to hold a wound open to thoroughly irrigate it, the wound should probably be taped shut. *Note:* After cleaning, wounds that gape more than ½ inch should not be closed in the field but instead dressed and evacuated for closure by a physician. When closing a wound and hair gets in the way, you can carefully clip the hair short, but it should not be shaved. If you have tincture of benzoin compound, smear a line along both sides of the wound. Benzoin is an irritant, however, so take care to keep it out of the wound. Let the benzoin dry for about thirty seconds. Benzoin's stickiness will help keep the closure strips in place. Touch the closure strips only on their ends to avoid contamination. Apply one end of one strip to one side of the wound and another to the opposite side. By using the opposing strips as handles, you can pull the wound edges together, pulling the skin as close as possible to where it should lie naturally—not too tight, not too loose. Use as many strips as needed to entirely close the wound.

Note: Large, dirty wounds; wounds, that expose bones, tendons, or ligaments; and wounds caused by animal bites should be left open. They are difficult to clean well enough to prevent infection. After irrigation, cover these wounds with sterile gauze. Exceptionally dirty wounds should be packed open with moist, sterile gauze and covered with dry gauze to allow them to drain until a physician can be consulted.

WOUND DRESSING

The *dressing* is the primary covering of a wound. It works best if it is sterile, nonadherent, porous, resistant to bacterial invasion, and easy to use. Wounds heal faster with less scarring if they are kept slightly moist with an antibiotic ointment or with a dressing that holds in the body's moisture, such as a microthin film dressing. Film dressings have the added advantage of being see-through and water repelling. The dressing should completely cover the wound and ideally extend ½ inch or so beyond the wound's edge. If you use a microthin film dressing, do *not* use an ointment. Dressing, ideally, should be changed at least once every twenty-four hours, although transparent film dressings may be left in place until healing is complete.

The function of a *bandage* is to fix, protect, and further assist the dressing. It can be conforming gauze, tape, elastic wraps, clean cotton strips, or improvised out of anything available. The usefulness of a bandage is handicapped if it is too loose and dangerous if it is too tight. Do not hide rings or anything that could cut off circulation if swelling occurs. Check bandages often.

NOTES ON SPECIFIC WOUNDS

Bruises (contusions): Usually no problem, but if they are big and over organs, watch for signs of internal bleeding (see "Shock"). *Note:* Large bruises will freeze faster than healthy skin in extreme cold.

Lacerations (cuts): Should be taped shut if they gape open (see above).

Avulsions (flaps): Lift up the flap to irrigate thoroughly underneath. Use closure strips to hold it in place (see above).

Amputations: Save the amputated part, preferably wrapped in moist, sterile gauze and then sealed in a clean plastic bag and placed in ice water.

Impalements: Generally do not remove them unless they are very loose. Carefully stabilize the object in place. An exception is an object through the cheek because it may threaten the airway.

Abrasions (scrapes): Scrubbing is the best way to clean these shallow, dirty wounds. Use of an anesthetic cleansing pad prior to scrubbing can ease the pain a little, but be prepared for a patient's reaction to the discomfort of scrubbing the wound's surface. Scrub with a gauze pad and soap and water or with an impregnated sponge, e.g., Green Soap Sponge. Follow scrubbing with irrigation. Apply a thin layer of antibiotic ointment, then a dressing and bandage.

WOUND INFECTION

Any wound may show signs of mild infection: pain, redness, swelling, and a little light-colored pus. These wounds should be recleaned, redressed, and monitored closely. Monitor for signs of serious infection: 1) increasing pain, redness, and swelling—the primary indicators; 2) increasing heat at the site; 3) more than a little pus; 4) appearance of red streaks just under the skin near the wound; and 5) systemic fever. If you see signs of serious infection, reopen the wound and let it drain. You may need to encourage the process with soaks in water as hot as the patient can tolerate. Pack the wound with moist, sterile gauze to keep it draining and dress it with dry, sterile gauze. Wet-to-dry dressings encourage draining.

Reclean and repack the wound twice a day, if possible. And start looking for a doctor.

EVACUATION GUIDELINES

Evacuate anyone with a wound that cannot be closed in the field. Evacuate *rapidly* anyone with a wound that 1) is heavily contaminated, 2) opens a joint space, 3) involves tendons or ligaments, 4) was caused by an animal bite, 5) is deep and on the face, 6) involves an impalement, and 7) was caused by a crushing injury.

Evacuate anyone with an infected wound that does not improve within twelve to twenty-four hours. Evacuate *rapidly* anyone with signs and symptoms of a serious infection.

11. Burns

Burns are among the most painful and emotionally distressing of injuries. Even relatively minor burns may disrupt the wilderness experience of an individual or an expedition.

INITIAL CARE

1. Remove the patient from the source of the burn.

2. Stop the burning process. The faster the better—within thirty seconds, if possible. Burns can continue to injure

tissue for a surprisingly long time after removal from the source. No first aid will be effective until the burning process has stopped. Smother flames, if appropriate, then cool the burn with water. Do not try to remove tar or melted plastic.

3. Be immediately suspicious of possible airway complications with burns to the face and/or neck, soot in the nose and/or mouth, singed facial hair, and a dry cough.

EVALUATION OF THE BURN

Specific burn treatment depends on your assessment of the depth and extent of the injury. Even though this assessment may be rough, it will be your basis for deciding how the patient will be managed, whether evacuation is required, and, if so, how urgently.

Depth

Superficial burns: Skin is red, painful, and swollen. Patient can almost always stay in the backcountry.

Partial-thickness burns: Skin is red, painful, swollen, and blisters form, sometimes more than an hour after cooling. Consider evacuating the patient (see below).

Full-thickness burns: Skin is painless with no blisters—although partial-thickness burns may surround full-thickness burns—and pale or charred. Evacuate the patient.

Extent

Use the rule of palmar surface: The palmar surface—inner surface of palm and fingers—equals about 1 percent of the total body surface area, or TBSA. The more TBSA burned, of course, the more serious the injury (see below).

Note: Do not underestimate the value of *pain* in addition to depth and extent as burn-assessment tools. If the patient is in a lot of pain, that is an indication of the need for a physician's care.

TREATMENT FOR THE BURNED PATIENT

1. Gently wash the burn with slightly warm water and mild soap. Pat dry.

2. Remove the skin from blisters that have popped open (but do not open blisters). Gently wipe away serum and obvious dirt.

3. Dress the burn with a thin layer of antibiotic ointment.

4. Cover the burn with a gauze pad or a thin layer of roll gauze, or apply clean clothing. Covering wounds reduces pain and evaporative losses.

5. Do not pack wounds or patient in ice.

6. Elevate burned extremities to minimize swelling. Swelling retards healing and encourages infection. Get the

patient, as much as possible, to gently and regularly move burned areas.

7. Ibuprofen is probably the best over-the-counter painkiller for burn pain (including sunburn).

8. If you have no ointment, no dressings, and/or no skill, leave the burn alone. The burn's surface will dry into a scablike covering that provides a significant amount of protection.

9. Keep the patient warm.

10. Keep the patient well hydrated.

Note: When evacuation is imminent, do not redress or re-examine the injury. But if evacuation is distant, redress twice a day by removing old dressings (you may have to soak off old dressings with clean, tepid water), rewashing (removing the old ointment), and putting on a clean covering.

EVACUATION GUIDELINES

Evacuate all patients with serious burns to the face, neck, hands, feet, armpits, or groin, as well as all patients with full-thickness burns. *Rapidly* evacuate all patients with burns threatening the airway, with partial- or full-thickness circumferential burns, and with blisters and/or full-thickness burns covering 15 percent TBSA.

12. Musculoskeletal Injuries

Musculoskeletal injuries, as presented here, involve damage to muscles and bones as well as damage to ligaments and, perhaps, tendons and cartilage—although in the field you may not be able to determine exactly what body part is injured.

STRAINS

Strains are overstretched muscles and/or tendons that attach muscles to bones. They can range from mildly annoying to debilitating. A strain can be used within the limits of pain—in other words, if it hurts, do not do it. RICE can be helpful (see "Sprains" below).

If a strain involves *low back pain* and comes on suddenly, apply cold for twenty to thirty minutes, several times a day, for the first forty-eight hours. If the pain grew gradually, heat usually works best. After two days, heat is usually best in both cases. Patient should rest in a side position or on the back with high padding beneath the knees. A nonsteroidal anti-inflammatory drug (e.g., ibuprofen) or acetaminophen is recommended. Massages may help. Reasons to evacuate a back-strained patient include: 1) The pain (or numbness) begins to radiate into the hip and/or thigh or all the way down a leg, 2) the pain remains strong even when the injured area is at rest, 3) the pain started as a result of illness, and

4) the pain came on sharply after a fall from a height or a sudden jolting stop.

SPRAINS

Sprains are injuries to ligaments, the bands holding bones to bones at joints, and can vary from simple overstretching to complete tears. Unlike fractures that mend strong and strains that heal well, a sprain may come back to haunt you the rest of your life, especially if you treat it improperly. What is really unfortunate about sprains is that they do not hurt as much as they should. Pain would encourage sensible action. Sensible action involves proper first aid and adequate support for the injury.

   Note: Strains and sprains, especially where a joint is involved, are often impossible to differentiate. Differentiation, however, is not required. They are treated the same.

   First aid is *RICE: r*est, *i*ce, *c*ompression, and *e*levation. But RICE should be applied *after* an initial evaluation of the injury. The primary goal of the evaluation is to *determine if the injury is usable or not.* Get the patient at rest and relaxed— and take a look at the injury. Look for deformities and rapid swelling and discoloration. Have the patient actively move the joint and evaluate the amount of pain involved. Move the joint more aggressively with your hands and evaluate the pain response. Finally, if the joint appears usable, have the patient test it with his or her body weight. A usable injury can be, well, used. An unusable injury will require a splint (see below).

Whether the injury is usable or unusable, have the patient stay off the injury (rest) for the first half hour while you reduce its temperature (ice) as much as possible without freezing the skin. Crushed ice works best. It conforms to the shape of the anatomy involved. Do *not* put ice directly on skin—put it in a plastic bag and wrap it in a shirt or sock. If ice is not available, soak the injury in cold water, or use a chemical cold packs, or (during warmer months) wrap the joint in wet cotton and let evaporation cool the damaged area. Compression (C) requires an elastic wrap. Wrap the elastic snugly but not tightly enough to cut off healthy circulation, and wrap from below the injury toward the heart. Elevation (E) refers to keeping the injury higher than the patient's heart. After twenty to thirty minutes of RICE, remove the treatment and let the joint warm naturally for ten

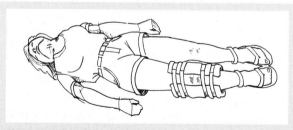

Figure 9. Walking knee splint

to fifteen minutes before use. (*Note:* The injury will heal faster if RICE is repeated three to four times a day until pain and swelling subside.)

The patient will benefit also from adequate hydration and regular use of a painkilling drug such as ibuprofen. After RICE, a splint that allows the joint to function will aid the patient.

A walking splint for the knee should hold the knee in place without putting pressure on the kneecap. Place a pad behind the knee within the splint to keep the knee slightly flexed.

Ankle taping should be applied firmly but not tight enough to cut off circulation and as wrinkle free as possible.

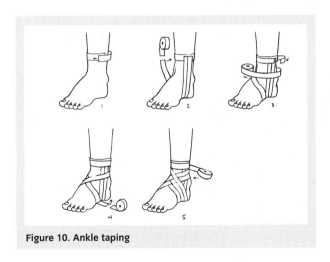

Figure 10. Ankle taping

The tape should be applied as 1) "stirrups" to pull the bones of the ankle together bottom to top, and 2) "figures of eight" to pull the bones of the ankle together side to side.

FRACTURES

Sometimes the assessment of a broken bone is simple: Bones stick out through the skin, or joints are created where no joint should exist. Without the obvious, and without an X-ray, rescuers can base an assessment on common sense and a good *LAF* at the patient. The goal, once again, is to determine whether or not the injury is usable.

L stands for **look.** Remove or cut away clothing carefully and take a look at the site of the injury. (In cold weather reduce "cutting away" to a minimum.) Is there discoloration and swelling? Does the patient move the injury easily or guard it jealously? Compare the injured side to the uninjured side. Does it *look* broken?

A stands for **ask.** Ask the patient: "How did the injury occur?" (High-speed impacts cause more damage than low-speed impacts.) "Do you think you have something broken?" (The patient is often right.) "How bad does it hurt?" (Surrounding muscle spasms create pain and give evidence of the seriousness of the injury.)

F stands for **feel.** Gently touch the damaged area. Does the patient react to your touch? ("Ouch!") Does it feel like the muscles are spasming? Does it feel unstable? Is there "point tenderness"—one particular spot that hurts noticeably more when touched? These are indications of a fracture.

Check for *circulation, sensation,* and *motion (CSM)* beyond the site of the injury. Loss of a pulse, numbness, tingling, and inability to move are signs of loss of normal blood flow and loss of normal nerve messages—serious complications with a fracture. After splinting, check CSM often to assure circulation is not cut off by wraps that are too tight.

Remember: Patients, whether a bone is actually broken or not, will usually benefit from RICE and a painkilling drug.

Splinting

The general rule is: *When in doubt, splint!* A splint should immobilize the broken bones, prevent further injury, and maximize patient comfort until a medical facility can be reached. To do this best, a splint needs to be made of 1) something to pad the injury comfortably, and 2) something rigid enough to provide support. Padding should fill all the spaces within the system to prevent movement of the injury. *Avoid the void!* In addition, a splint should be long enough to immobilize the joints above and below a broken bone or to immobilize the bones above and below an injured joint.

Splints should immobilize the injury in the position of function, or as close to position of function as possible. Functional positions include the 1) spine, including neck and pelvis, straight with padding in the small of the back; 2) legs almost straight with padding behind the knees for slight flexion;

3) feet at 90 degrees to legs; 4) arms flexed to cross the heart; and 5) hands in a functional curve with padding in the palms.

In choosing materials for splinting, you are only limited by imagination: sleeping bags, foamlite pads (they can be cut to fit the problem), extra clothing, or soft debris from the forest floor stuffed into extra clothing. For rigidity there are items such as sticks, tent poles, ski poles, and ice axes, Crazy Creek Chairs, and internal and external pack frames. Lightweight commercial splints are available as additions to your first-aid kit (e.g., Sam Splint or wire splints). Splints can be secured in place with things like bandannas, strips of clothing, pack straps, belts, and rope. Useful items in your first-aid kit for securing splints include tape, elastic wraps, and roll gauze. Large triangular bandages are helpful in creating slings and swathes.

Specific Fractures

Jaw fractures can be held in place with a wide wrap that goes around the head. Be sure the wrap can be removed quickly if the patient feels like vomiting.

Collarbone (clavicle) fractures can be secured with a sling and swathe. Slings can be made from triangular bandages

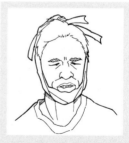

Figure 11. Jaw splint

or improvised by lifting the tail of the patient's shirt up over the arm on the injured side and safety-pinning it in place. Be sure the sling lifts the elbow to take pressure off the shoulder.

Lower arm (radius and/or ulna) fractures (including wrist and hand) can be secured to a well-padded rigid support and then held in a sling and swathe. Place a roll of something soft in the hand to keep it in position of function. If bones of the hand are damaged, be sure to secure the hand well to the splint with lots of padding.

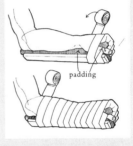

padding

Figure 12. Lower arm splint

Fingers that are broken can be secured to nearby healthy fingers with padding between the fingers.

Upper arm (humerus) fractures can be placed in a sling and swathe. Leaving the elbow free sometimes eases the pain. Secure the broken bone to the patient's chest wall with a wide soft wrap.

Rib fractures can be protected by supporting the arm on the injured side with a sling and swathe. Do *not* wrap a band snugly around the patient's chest. *Do* encourage the patient to take deep breaths regularly, even if it hurts, to keep the lungs clear. Be sure to watch the patient for increasing difficulty breathing (see "Chest Injuries").

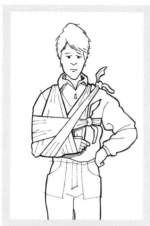
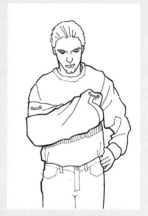

Figure 13. Sling and swathe   **Figure 14. Shirt as sling**

Pelvic fractures should include a conforming wrap secured around the patient's pelvis below the navel. The wrap need only be 4 to 5 inches wide. Secure the entire patient on a rigid litter before attempting a carryout. Be sure to watch the patient for signs of shock due to internal bleeding common with pelvic fractures.

Hip fractures should involve gently straightening the leg on the affected side and securing the legs comfortably to each other with padding between the legs. As with a fractured pelvis, a hip fracture requires evacuating the patient on a rigid litter.

Lower leg (tibia and/or fibula) fractures (including the ankle and foot) can be secured on a well-padded rigid support that includes immobilization of the ankle and foot. Closed cell foam sleeping pads, Crazy Creek Chairs, and Therm-a-Rest pads (deflated and then blown up after being secured in place) make excellent lower leg splints. Pad behind the knee for comfort.

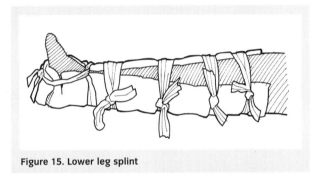

Figure 15. Lower leg splint

Thigh (femur) fractures may be splinted by immobilizing the entire leg with adequate padding and rigid support—but femurs are better treated with a splint that provides traction to the fracture. To manage a broken femur best, the leg should get gentle, manual traction-in-line as soon as possible. Prompt manual traction 1) prevents further injury from movement or massive spasms of the large thigh muscles, 2) reduces bleeding into the thigh, which can be severe even without an open wound, and 3) reduces pain, which can be extreme. *Maintain manual traction until a traction splint is in place.* Splinting a fractured femur requires a device that maintains traction on the leg. Commercial products are available (such as the Kendrick Traction Device—KTD for short), but such a device can be improvised in the field. Several methods of improvising traction exist. Here's one:

1. One rescuer should hold traction while a second rescuer gathers material.

2. Create a fixation splint beneath or around the patient's thigh.

3. Create a hitch or harness at the ankle on the injured side.

4. A shaft (stick, ski pole, paddle, tent pole, etc.) about 6 to 8 inches longer than the patient's leg is secured to the outside of the patient's leg at hip level.

5. Using a rope, cord, or strong cloth, apply traction between the ankle hitch and the outer end of the shaft via a trucker's hitch until the mechanical traction is equal to or greater than the manual traction. (The patient is a good judge of the amount of traction.)

6. Secure the system, backing up knots and padding all possible pressure points.

7. An evacuation via a rigid litter, as soon as possible, is required.

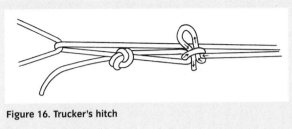

Figure 16. Trucker's hitch

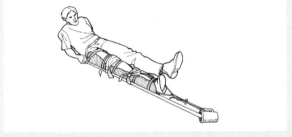

Figure 17. Traction splint

Complicated Fractures

An *angulated fracture* (angles in bones in the wrong place)
needs to be realigned to normal anatomical position. Pull gentle traction on the broken bone *along the line in which it lies*.
This relaxes the muscles and reduces the pain, allowing you to
move the broken bone slowly and gently back into normal

alignment. The sooner this movement takes place the better. Do *not* use force. Do *not* continue if the patient complains of increasing pain. Once the bone is aligned, splint as usual. If alignment cannot be achieved, splint as best you can.

An *open fracture* is indicated by an open wound over the fracture. Bones may or may not be visible. All open fractures should be seen by a physician as soon as possible. The wound should be irrigated and dressed appropriately (see "Wound and Wound Infection Management"), and the bone should be splinted. If bone ends stick out of the wound, and if the doctor is more than four to six hours away, 1) clean the wound and bone ends without scrubbing, 2) apply gentle traction-in-line to the fracture and pull the bone ends back under the skin, 3) dress the wound, and 4) splint. Infection is on the way, but bones live longer inside the body.

DISLOCATIONS

With a dislocation the bone ends in a joint are no longer properly aligned. The patient typically experiences pain in the joint and a loss of normal range of motion. The joint looks "wrong." If a doctor is nearby, splint the joint to stabilize it in the position found. When the doctor is far away, attempt to reduce (relocate) the dislocation before splinting.

Work quickly but calmly. Typically the sooner a reduction is attempted, the easier it is on patient and rescuer. Encourage the patient to relax as much as possible, with special concentration on relaxing the injured joint. Place yourself in a position that will allow you to pull gentle traction-in-line. With a firm grip on both sides of the dislocated joint (sometimes a team of two rescuers works better), pull *along the lines in which the bones lie*. Under gentle traction, move the bones toward normal alignment. *Do not use force*. It may cause pain, but *stop if pain increases dramatically*. Once reduced, the injury should be splinted (see above). Most patients will benefit from RICE and a painkilling drug.

Note: The reduction of dislocations falls outside the scope of practice of most first-aid providers and should not be attempted by outdoor leaders without prior permission from a medical advisor.

Specific Dislocations

Jaw dislocations can be reduced by wrapping something soft around your thumbs (e.g., gauze), reaching into the patient's mouth, and pressing down and forward with your thumbs on the back molars.

Cervical spine (neck) dislocations qualify as a possible spinal cord injury and should be treated as such (see "Spinal Injuries").

Shoulder dislocations are among the most common. There are several ways to reduce a dislocated shoulder. Here is one with a high rate of success:

1. The patient may be standing or sitting but lying down usually works best.

2. Pull gentle traction-in-line, pulling along the line in which the patient's arm on the dislocated side lies. Keep the patient's arm flexed, and pull from the elbow.

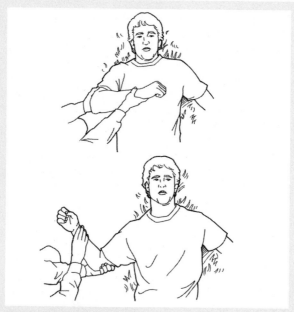

Figure 18. Shoulder relocation

3. Under traction, move the arm away from the body while simultaneously rotating the arm outward, toward the baseball-throwing position.

4. If reduction does not occur, and the arm is still under traction, move the arm to the side of the chest.

5. If reduction does not occur, bring the arm across the body while simultaneously rotating the arm inward into the pledge-of-allegiance position.

Here is another technique to treat shoulder dislocations, but you might have a long wait for reduction:

1. Have the patient lie prone (face down) across a rock or log with the arm on the injured side dangling down vertically.

2. With a soft cloth, tie something of about fifteen pounds' weight to the dangling wrist.

3. Wait.

Wrist dislocations are usually associated with a fracture of the wrist. Reduction is typically simple. Splint well.

Finger dislocations are also common. Keeping the injured finger partially flexed, pull on the end while gently pressing the dislocated joint back into place with your other thumb. Tape the injured finger to a neighbor with a gauze pad between them. Do *not* tape directly over the joint itself.

Knee dislocations usually leave the knee useless for walking. Applying gentle traction, move the leg to normal alignment, splint securely, and figure out how to carry the patient.

Kneecap (patella) dislocations are typically easy to reduce. Apply gentle traction to the leg to straighten it out. Sometimes the kneecap pops back into place when the leg is straightened. If it does not, massage the thigh and push the kneecap gently back into normal alignment with your hand. Wearing a splint that does not put pressure on the kneecap (see the walking knee splint shown in fig. 9), the patient can usually walk out.

Ankle dislocations usually involve fractured bones and are easy to reduce. Reduction can usually be achieved by taking hold of the patient's toes and lifting until the weight of the leg acts as countertraction. A gentle pull on the heel may be required. Splint well.

Toe dislocations are treated the same as fingers.

EVACUATION GUIDELINES

With a usable injury, the patient's degree of discomfort will determine more than anything the need to evacuate the patient. Evacuate all patients with unusable injuries and with first-time dislocations (except perhaps dislocations of the outer joints of the fingers and toes). Evacuate *rapidly* all open fractures and injuries that create a decrease in CSM beyond the injury.

13. Hypothermia

Hypothermia is a lowering of the body's core temperature to a point where normal brain and/or muscle function is impaired. This condition may be mild, moderate, or life-threateningly severe.

SIGNS AND SYMPTOMS OF HYPOTHERMIA

Mild: *Shivering,* inability to perform complex tasks (fumbles); confusion, apathy, and sluggish thinking (grumbles); slurred speech (mumbles); and altered gait (stumbles)—sometimes referred to collectively as "the umbles."

Moderate: Worsening of "the umbles" and *uncontrollable violent shivering*.

Severe: *Shivering stops;* patient displays increasing muscle rigidity, stupor progressing to coma, decreasing pulse and respirations to the point where they are undetectable (but still present!).

MANAGEMENT OF HYPOTHERMIA

Management can be divided, for simplicity, into two categories: 1) treatment for mild and moderate hypothermia, and 2) treatment for severe hypothermia.

The *mild-moderate hypothermia* patient is still trying to warm up internally. The patient can talk, eat, and shiver.

Change the environment so the heat being produced internally is not lost. Get the patient out of wet clothes and into something dry, out of wind and cold, and into some kind of shelter, even if the only shelter available is the protection of waterproof, windproof clothing. Cover the patient's head and neck. If the patient can take food and drink, give her or him simple carbohydrates to stoke the inner fire. Fluids are more important than solids to a cold person. A warm (not hot), sweet drink will add a tiny bit of heat and a lot of simple sugar for energy. Even cold fluids are better than no fluids. If the patient can still exercise easily, you may keep him or her moving after initial treatment. If the patient cannot exercise easily, do all you can to encourage entrapment of inner heat production: Insulate the patient from the ground, bundle in dry insulation, snuggle with warm people, place hot water bottles in the hands or at the feet (but not against naked skin), use chemical heat packs as you would hot water bottles—and wait until the patient returns to normal.

The *severe hypothermia* patient is semiconscious or unconscious and has stopped shivering. She or he has lost the ability to rewarm. *Handle the patient gently*—roughness can overload a cold heart and stop it. Perform rescue breathing for five to fifteen minutes prior to any movement. Remove the person's clothing and bundle her or him up in as much dry insulation as possible. Insulate well from the ground. Wrap hot water bottles or heat packs in a dry sock or shirt and place them appropriately: over the heart (with the hands over the heat source, if possible), armpits, and groin—in that order. Finish with a vapor barrier—a tent fly, a sheet of plastic, garbage bags—something to trap any heat still left in the patient. The final product is a cocoon, a "hypothermia wrap" open only to the mouth and nose. Do *not* try to force food or drink. Treat for severe hypothermia even if the patient appears dead. *No patient is dead, as far as you are concerned, unless the patient is warm and dead*. Call for help immediately—do *not* try to evacuate the patient by any means other than gentle.

PREVENTION OF HYPOTHERMIA

It is far easier to maintain core temperature than to regain core temperature. Therefore:

1. Wear clothing that retains body heat even when wet.
2. Stay dry by wearing layers of clothing, taking off layers before sweating starts, and adding them back before chilling occurs.
3. Drink lots of water.
4. Eat lots, especially carbohydrates.
5. Maintain a pace that prevents overexertion. Rest often.
6. In a group, watch each other for signs of hypothermia. Treat early, and if one person is treated, treat everyone.

EVACUATION GUIDELINES

Evacuate *rapidly* and with extreme gentleness anyone with severe hypothermia.

14. Local Cold Injury: Frozen and Nonfrozen

Localized tissue damage from exposure to cold may involve frozen tissue (frostbite) or nonfrozen tissue (immersion foot).

FROSTBITE

Frostbite is localized freezing of tissue, and it often walks frigid hand-in-hand with hypothermia. Proper treatment of local cold injury can save near-frozen tissue and reduce the extent of already frozen tissue.

Partial-Thickness Frostbite

When this occurs, skin is pale and numb, but it moves when you press on it. Begin passive warming immediately. In the field cover the cold body part with warm body parts. Cover your nose with your warm hand, stick your cold hand against your warm stomach, put your cold toes against the warm stomach of a friend. Do *not* rub the cold skin. Do *not* place cold skin near a hot heat source because numb tissue is very susceptible to heat injury. Give ibuprofen, if available, and lots of water to drink.

Skin that looks okay after warming is usually okay. If blisters form after warming, a physician should be consulted as soon as possible in most cases (see below). In the meantime, two things should be remembered: 1) Leave the bubble intact. It protects the underlying tissue and creates less of a chance for infection. 2) Blisters freeze quickly, multiplying the damage. Be careful to prevent freezing by protecting the injured tissue from exposure to cold.

Full-Thickness Frostbite

Skin is pale and numb—and hard. A patient can still travel on frozen feet, making an evacuation speedier. Although the frozen parts benefit from thawing as soon as possible, normal field conditions often make warming of deep frostbite impractical, and the patient overall is likely to do better with a faster evacuation.

If refreezing is unlikely, and you have the means available, you can best treat full-thickness frostbite by rapid warming in water of approximately 104 to 108 degrees F (40 to 42 degrees C). Too hot and heat damage occurs. Too cold and thawing is too slow for maximum benefit. Warming is usually accomplished in thirty to forty minutes, but it is better to err on the side of caution and warm longer than necessary rather than less than necessary. Place soft cotton between thawed digits, but otherwise contact with anything should be avoided. Pain is often intense, and painkillers should be started prior to thawing. Aspirin started as soon as possible seems to reduce the extent of damage to tissue. Without aspirin, ibuprofen may be used. Keep the patient well hydrated. Prevention of refreezing is of paramount importance. Find a doctor as soon as possible.

Prevention of Frostbite

Follow the same guidelines that prevent hypothermia. Avoid snug clothing that restricts circulation, especially on the feet and hands. Wear clothing appropriate for cold weather, e.g., insulated boots and mittens rather than gloves. Be careful to protect your skin from wind and from contact with cold metal and cold gasoline. Avoid alcohol and tobacco. If your toes hurt from the cold, rejoice—and stop and warm them before they go numb and possibly suffer permanent injury.

NONFREEZING COLD INJURY

When tissue remains cold and wet a long time but never freezes, you may suffer a nonfreezing cold injury known as immersion foot (although the problem can occur on hands as well). The primary symptom is pain, but the foot may appear pale or mottled. Follow the treatment recommendations for partial-thickness frostbite. Prevent immersion foot by starting each day with dry socks and changing into dry socks after a day of travel.

EVACUATION GUIDELINES
Evacuate 1) patients with blisters (unless the blisters are filled with clear fluid and are no more than the size of a quarter and can be kept from refreezing), 2) patients with full-thickness frostbite, and 3) patients in pain that cannot be reduced to acceptable limits.

15. Heat Illness

"Heat illness" describes a range of problems associated with a rise in air temperature—everything from the fatigue of heat exhaustion to the life threat of heat stroke. In addition to rising temperatures, other factors increase your risk of heat illness: 1) high humidity; 2) being overweight; 3) being very young or very old; 4) being unaccustomed to heat; 5) taking certain drugs, such as antihistamines (consult your physician); and 6) being dehydrated—often the most important factor.

HEAT EXHAUSTION
The patient has been exercising and sweating out water and salt and now feels very tired. Skin may appear pale or flushed

and sweaty, and the patient complains of a headache, per-haps nausea, and sometimes vomiting. Thirst is usual, as well as a decreased urine output. Dizziness may strike when the patient stands quickly. An elevated heart rate and respiratory rate are common.

The problem is a volume problem—not enough water inside the patient—and it is typically not serious. Core tem-perature may have risen a few degrees or, more often, not at all. The cure is suggested by the name of the condition: Exhaustion calls for rest, preferably in a cool, shady spot. Replace lost fluids with water and lost salt by adding a pinch to a liter of water or by munching salty snacks. Oral rehydra-tion salts or a sports drink will work. Do *not* use salt tablets—they are too concentrated. To increase the rate of cooling, the patient may be wet down and fanned. A drowsy patient may be allowed to sleep. When the patient feels okay, the backcountry adventure may be continued.

HEAT CRAMPS

Associated with heat exhaustion are heat cramps, most com-monly occurring in the large muscles of the legs and some-times extending up into the abdomen. Though the discomfort may be great, the problem is rarely serious. Treat-ment includes rest, gentle stretching and massage, and drinking water, preferably with a pinch of salt added per liter or with a salty snack. Oral rehydration salts or a sports drink will work. Once feeling well, the patient may continue. But if the cramps return, the sufferer should take the rest of the day off. Overworking depleted muscles can lead to a serious injury.

HEAT STROKE

Heat stroke occurs when a patient is producing core heat faster than it can be shed. The patient may be overexerting and/or seriously dehydrated, and the core temperature rises to 105 degrees F (40.6 degrees C) or more. Disorientation and bizarre personality changes are common signs. Skin turns hot and red and sometimes (but far from always) dry. Look for a fast heart rate, fast breathing, and complaints of a headache.

Heat stroke is a temperature problem. The patient is too hot inside. Once a human brain gets that hot, it is a *true emergency*, and only rapid cooling will save the patient. Take off any heat-retaining clothes and drench the patient with water. Concentrate cooling efforts on the head and neck. Cold packs may be used on the neck, armpits, groin, and hands and feet. Fan the patient constantly to increase evaporation. Massage the limbs to encourage cooler blood to return to the core. When or if the patient is able to accept and drink cool water, give it. Do *not* give fever-reducing drugs. The patient must see a doctor as soon as possible, even if she or he appears to have recovered. During evacuation, a careful watch on the patient should be maintained. Relapses are common.

HYPONATREMIA

It is possible to drink too much water—if you are not eating. Salt loss in sweat exceeding salt intake plus water intake exceeding water loss equals lowered sodium level in the blood. When blood sodium gets too low, you have a case of hyponatremia.

Common complaints include headache, weakness, fatigue, lightheadedness, muscle cramps, nausea with or without vomiting, sweaty skin, normal core temperature, normal or slightly elevated pulse and respirations, and a bit of anxiety. Sound familiar? Yep, it sounds like heat exhaustion. But if you treat it like heat exhaustion—just add water—you are harming the hyponatremia patient. More severe symptoms of hyponatremia include a patient who is disoriented, irritable, and combative—which gives the problem a more common name: water intoxication. Untreated, the ultimate result will be seizures, coma, and death.

Heat-exhausted patients typically have a low output of yellowish urine (urinating every six to eight hours) combined with thirst. Hyponatremia patients have urinated recently and the urine was probably clear. Hyponatremia patients will also claim to have been drinking a lot of water, and they deny thirst.

Patients with mild to moderate symptoms and a normal

mental status may be treated in the field: Rest in shade with no fluid intake and a gradual intake of salty foods while the kidneys reestablish a sodium balance. Once a patient develops hunger and thirst combined with normal urine output, the problem is solved. Restriction of fluids for someone who is well hydrated, fortunately, is harmless. Concerning patients with an altered mental status there is no question: They demand rapid evacuation to a medical facility.

PREVENTION OF HEAT ILLNESS

1. Stay well hydrated. Urine output should be clear and relatively copious, an indication of adequate hydration. Water is probably best to drink, and sports drinks are okay. Remember, it is possible to drink too much water. Avoid alcohol and caffeinated drinks.

2. Munch on lightly salted snacks.

3. Wear baggy, loosely woven clothing that allows evaporation of sweat. Keep your head covered.

4. Keep yourself fit, and allow time for acclimatization when you are new to a hot environment. Go slow the first few days, and avoid the hottest times of day.

5. Beware drugs that increase your risk of heat illness, including alcohol and antihistamines.

6. Rest often in the shade.

EVACUATION GUIDELINES

Evacuate *rapidly* anyone who has an altered mental status due to heat or hyponatremia.

16. Lightning

The awesome power of a lightning strike may produce several types of patients: 1) nonbreathing patients who may respond to rescue breathing; 2) pulseless, nonbreathing patients who may respond to CPR; 3) the battered around who have sustained treatable injuries; and 4) the stunned who are not really hurt at all. After a lightning strike, assess and treat first those patients who appear dead—they might be recoverable.

To maximize your safety, follow these guidelines:

1. **Know local weather patterns.** Lightning storms, in general, tend to roll in quickly in summer afternoons.

2. **Plan turnaround times** in lightning zones, and stick to the plan.

3. **Monitor approaching storms.** Lightning can strike miles ahead of a storm. Five seconds between the flash of lightning and the boom of thunder indicates the storm is 1 mile away (three seconds indicates 1 kilometer). When the storm is 6 miles away, you should be in a safe spot.

4. **Find a safe spot.**
   Avoid high places,
   high objects, metal
   objects, open places,
   low places, open
   bodies of water
   (especially the shore-
   line), shallow caves,
   overhangs, places
   obviously struck in
   the past, and long
   conductors (such as
   fences). Seek uniform
   cover, e.g., low rolling
   hills or trees of about
   the same size, deep

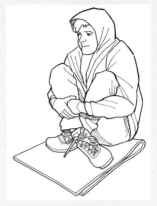

Figure 19. Lightning protection
position

dry caves, buildings, or cars with the windows rolled up.

5. **Assume a safe position when outdoors.** Squat or
   sit in a tight position on insulating material. Spread
   groups out, but try to keep everyone in sight.

6. **Pick safe campsites.**

7. **Be sure everyone in a group understands the
   lightning plan.**

EVACUATION GUIDELINES

Evacuate all patients who have been struck by lightning, even if they appear to be okay, soon after the injury. Serious problems sometimes develop later.

17. Submersion Incidents

No backcountry situation has more inherent danger for rescuers than one in which someone is drowning. Follow these guidelines for getting the drowning person safely out of the water:

1. **Reach** to the victim with your hand or foot, clothing, a stick, a paddle, or anything that allows you to remain safely on land or in a boat.

2. **Throw** something that floats to the victim.

3. **Row** to the victim or access the person in some sort of watercraft.

4. **Tow** the person to safety by throwing out a line and hauling him or her in.

5. **Go** if all else fails, and if you have been trained in swimming rescues, but go knowing you risk your own life.

Once the patient is safely out of the water, check for breathing. If necessary, begin rescue breathing (see "Airway

Obstructions and CPR"). There is no value in attempting to clear the patient's lungs of water, but be ready to roll him or her to clear the airway if water or vomit comes up. Check for signs of a beating heart, and begin CPR if necessary. All patients surviving a submersion incident should be warmed and evacuated as soon as possible, even if they appear fully recovered. Long-term problems often develop.

In *cold-water submersion incidents,* patients have been resuscitated after more than an hour of submersion, their spark of life probably kept alive by the rapid onset of hypothermia. In such cases do your best CPR, keep it going as long as possible, and hope for a miracle.

EVACUATION GUIDELINES

Evacuate anyone who was unconscious, no matter how short a time, during a submersion incident and anyone with signs and symptoms of respiratory problems after a submersion incident.

18. Bites and Stings

Creatures that bite or sting often cause a lot of aggravation and sometimes, though not often, pose a serious threat to the bitten or stung. In every instance you should know what to do.

SMALL INSECTS

The little biters (mosquitoes, blackflies, gnats, etc.) are the most bothersome but the least serious (except in countries where mosquitoes are still a primary source of disease). Bites can be reduced in number or prevented by these steps: 1) Wear clothing insects cannot bite through (*Note:* Lighter clothing colors appear to offer some repellent qualities). 2) Apply insect repellents on skin. Follow the directions on the product label carefully, especially with products containing deet. 3) Use permethrin products on clothing. You may also choose to avoid prime insect habitats, avoid being exposed during prime biting times (usually dawn and dusk), and sleep under mosquito netting or in a tent with mosquito netting. If you are bitten, a wipe with a sting-relief product (such as StingEze) can ease the itching. Antihistamines such as diphenhydramine (sold often as Benadryl) can reduce itching and swelling of more severe reactions.

BEES AND THEIR RELATIVES

The stinger left by honeybees should be removed as soon as possible. Any means to get it out is acceptable, despite thoughts to the contrary. Ice or cold packs on the stings from bees, wasps, yellow jackets, hornets, and fire ants will relieve pain and reduce swelling. Diphenhydramine may be given for itching and swelling. Watch the patient for an allergic reaction (see "Allergic Reactions/Anaphylaxis" in the "Medical Emergencies" section) to bees and their relatives.

SPIDERS

Shiny with an hourglass shape almost always on the abdomen, *black widows* have a bite that often goes unnoticed, but local pain and redness show up at the bite site usually within ten to sixty minutes. Pain from muscle cramping usually develops in the arm or leg bitten and in the abdomen and back. The pain may become incredibly severe. Sweating, chills, nausea, vomiting, and headache are not uncommon complaints. After cleaning the bite site, apply ice or cold packs to the site; this usually provides some relief. Painkilling drugs may be used, if available. Although most patients recover within twenty-four hours, evacuation to a doctor is strongly recommended, especially for children and the elderly.

Recluse (fiddleback) spiders have a violin shape on their back and a bite that usually produces local pain and blister formation within one to five hours. A bull's-eye of discoloration often surrounds the blister. The blister ruptures eventually, leaving a growing ulcer of skin destruction. Fever, chills, and weakness are usual. After cleaning the bite site, apply ice or cold packs to help relieve local pain. Painkilling drugs may be useful. If the blister ruptures, treat the open wound appropriately (see "Wound Management"). The patient should be seen by a physician for consideration of drug treatment to minimize damage.

SCORPIONS

Scorpion stings produce immediate pain and swelling. Sometimes the patient will develop numbness around the sting site. Ice or cold packs will reduce pain. Diphenhydramine can be given for swelling and itching. The patient will soon recover—except sometimes from the sting of *Centruroides*, a southwestern scorpion that may produce a systemic reaction characterized by unusual anxiety, sweating, salivation, gastrointestinal distress, and, most importantly, respiratory distress. No first aid specific to *Centruroides* stings is useful, and immediate evacuation should take place.

TICKS

Ticks may carry diseases that they can pass to humans. Insect repellents repel ticks, and ticks crawling around on your skin do not transmit diseases until they dig in and feed for hours to days. Careful "tick checks" should be performed at least twice a day in tick-infected country, and early removal of embedded ticks prevents the transmission of many diseases. Remove ticks gently with tweezers, without excess squeezing, by taking hold of the tick as near the skin as possible and pulling straight out. Any other removal method increases the risk of germ transmission. If a little of the patient's skin comes off with the tick, you have done well. If possible, save the tick for evaluation in case of illness in the patient. Wash the little wound. A swipe with an antiseptic may be useful. Watch the patient carefully for signs and symptoms of illness (e.g., rash, fever), which should send the patient to a doctor immediately.

SNAKES

In North America envenomations are almost always caused by either pit vipers or, far less frequently, coral snakes.

A *pit viper* (rattlesnake, water moccasin, or copperhead) bites with either or both retractable fangs, producing immediate local pain and swelling within approximately fifteen minutes. If swelling and pain are not present after thirty minutes, envenomation probably did not occur. With envenomation, blister formation and discoloration usually do occur and may lead to local skin destruction. Patients often report lip tingling and a funny taste in their mouth within an hour or so. Weakness, chills, and nausea may occur. Muscle twitching may result. Death is rare.

Coral snakes ("Bright red on yellow may kill a fellow" . . . or a woman) have to gnaw a few moments to deposit venom from nonretractable fixed fangs. Burning pain at the bite site is often followed by swelling and then pain, tingling, or numbness extending up from the bite—but these signs and symptoms may take up to twelve hours to develop. Serious systemic manifestations include difficulty speaking, swallowing, seeing, and breathing. Bites are far less common and far more dangerous.

After a Snakebite

1. Get away from the snake.

2. Remain as calm as possible.

3. Remove anything that might restrict circulation when swelling occurs, e.g., rings.

4. Gently wash the bite site.

5. Splint the bitten arm or leg, and keep the bite site on a level with the patient's heart.

6. Transport the patient to a doctor. Carrying the patient is best, but slow walking with a stable patient is acceptable.

7. Give acetaminophen for pain, but do not give nonsteroidal anti-inflammatory drugs such as ibuprofen and aspirin.

8. Do not use cold packs, tourniquets, cutting, sucking, or electrical shocks.

RABIES

The rabies virus is ultimately lethal once it reaches the brain. Highly suspect animals include bats, raccoons, foxes, skunks, the canines, the felines, and any mammal acting unnaturally.

Reduce the risk of any infection from any animal bite by immediate and aggressive wound cleaning and keeping the wound open to allow draining. In a suspect animal bite, seek medical attention as soon as possible for preventive drug therapy.

19. Altitude Illness

When you go higher in altitude, the amount of oxygen available in each breath grows lower. If you go too high too fast, problems may occur. For simplicity, these problems can be divided into two categories: mild and severe.

MILD ALTITUDE ILLNESS

Anyone coming from lower altitudes to 10,000 feet (3,048 meters), and often even at lower altitudes, may complain of acute mountain sickness (AMS): headache, unusual fatigue, nausea, loss of appetite, difficulty sleeping, unusual shortness of breath when exercising, and lassitude. The best treatment is: *Do not go up until the symptoms go down*. Stop ascending until the signs and symptoms go away. Light exercise is recommended, and stay hydrated and well fed. Acetazolamide may be used for treatment after symptoms appear, and this drug actually aids in acclimatization for many people. *Consult your physician,* and do *not* use acetazolamide if you are allergic to sulfa drugs. If the symptoms do not go down within two days, the patient should descend further. A descent of 2,000 feet (610 meters) usually brings relief of symptoms.

SEVERE ALTITUDE ILLNESS

Untreated mild illness may progress to severe. The most important early sign of this progression is often ataxia (loss of coordination). An ataxic patient cannot walk a straight line or stand straight with feet together and eyes closed. Ataxia typically indicates the patient is progressing into a severe form of altitude illness known as high-altitude cerebral edema (HACE): severe headache unrelieved by rest and medication, bizarre changes in personality, perhaps seizures and/or coma. Or severe altitude illness may show up as high-altitude pulmonary edema (HAPE): constant shortness of breath, chest pain, productive cough, and very fast heart rate. *Severely ill patients need to go down as soon as possible.* In addition to descent, the best treatment is supplemental oxygen. Treatment may also include the drug nifedipine (sold often as Procardia) for HAPE and the drug dexamethasone (sold often as Decadron) for HACE. *Consult your physician.* If descent is delayed, use of the Gamow Bag, a portable hyperbaric chamber that simulates descent, may save the patient's life. Do *not* use a Gamow Bag instead of descent.

PREVENTION OF ALTITUDE ILLNESS

1. Above 10,000 feet ascend no faster than your ability to acclimatize—an average of 1,000 to 1,500 feet (305 to 610 meters)/twenty-four hours of sleeping gain (in other words, sleep no more than 1,000 to 1,500 feet higher than the night before). You can climb high, but sleep low.

2. Drink plenty of water. It does not prevent sickness but is important for general health.

3. Exercise lightly every day.

4. Eat plenty of carbohydrate-rich low-fat foods. Above 16,000 feet (4,880 meters), a diet of at least 70 percent carbohydrates is recommended.

5. Avoid alcohol and sedatives.

6. Consult your physician about the uses of acetazolamide to prevent AMS, nifedipine to prevent HAPE, and dexamethasone to prevent AMS and HACE.

EVACUATION GUIDELINES

Evacuate (descend) with any sick patient who does not improve within forty-eight hours. Rapid descent and/or evacuation are recommended for all patients with signs and symptoms of severe altitude illness.

20. Medical Emergencies

When a patient complains of distress, and the problem is not related to trauma (forces from outside the body), you have a medical emergency (a problem related to disease or, you might say, a dysfunction inside the body).

ABDOMINAL PAIN

Anything from freeze-dried food to a raging appendicitis can cause complaints of abdominal pain. You may never know the source of the problem. For that reason it is recommended to evacuate any patient with abdominal pain if:

1. The pain is associated with the signs and symptoms of shock (see "Shock").

2. The pain persists for longer than twelve to twenty-four hours.

3. The pain localizes, and especially if the pain involves guarding (the patient voluntarily or involuntarily protects the area), tenderness, abdominal rigidity, and/or distention.

4. Blood appears in the vomit, feces, or urine. In vomit it may look like coffee grounds, in the stool black like tar, in the urine a reddish color.

5. Nausea, vomiting, and/or diarrhea persist for longer than twenty-four to seventy-two hours, especially if the patient is unable to stay well hydrated.

6. The pain is associated with a fever above 102 degrees F (38 degrees C).

7. The pain is associated with the signs and symptoms of pregnancy.

8. The patient complains of increased pain when a foot strikes the ground during walking.

If you decide the patient's condition is serious, evacuation should be gentle, with the patient in a position of greatest comfort, avoiding anything by mouth except small sips of cold water if the evacuation will be long.

ALLERGIC REACTIONS/ANAPHYLAXIS

Almost anything eaten, injected into, absorbed, or breathed in by a person can cause an allergic reaction. For simplicity, allergic reactions can be divided into two stages: mild and severe. Mild reactions are characterized by stuffy noses, itching, swelling, and/or hives. They can be treated in the field with an antihistamine, diphenhydramine (sold often as Benadryl) being a well-accepted choice.

A severe reaction, known as *anaphylaxis*, is a *true emergency*. Anaphylaxis may produce shock but is more often typified by extreme breathing difficulty, causing the sufferer to be unable to speak or to speak only in one- or two-word clusters. Swelling of the face, lips, tongue, and perhaps the hands and feet are to be expected. The patient's only salvation lies in an immediate injection of epinephrine (adrenaline). Injectable epinephrine is available commercially in spring-loaded syringes that function when pressed into the thigh. You may also be able to acquire epinephrine in small containers that require manually operated syringes to administer. Everyone who knows they are susceptible to severe allergic reactions should carry injectable epinephrine on all trips that take them far from a doctor. Leaders responsible for others in remote areas should consider carrying injectable epinephrine. Epinephrine can be ruined by extremes of cold and heat and needs to be protected from these extremes. A prescription is required. *Consult your physician*. Once the epinephrine opens the airway and allows the patient to swallow, an antihistamine, preferably diphenhydramine, should be given immediately. The patient should be 1) kept on the antihistamine, following the directions on the product's label, and 2) kept well hydrated during the evacuation to a hospital.

ASTHMA

Asthma is a recurring disease of the airway that causes swelling, increased mucus production, and spasms of the lower airway. Patients suffer moderate to severe respiratory difficulty during attacks. Air is often trapped in the lungs, causing the patient to breathe out slowly with difficulty and a wheezing sound. Treatment includes calm encouragement of the patient to relax and breathe with control. Asthmatics should carry inhalers at all times and pack extras on extended backcountry expeditions or trips to foreign countries. Assistance with the inhaler may be required. The medication in the inhaler must be sucked deep into the lungs to work. In extreme cases injected epinephrine may open the blocked airway of an asthmatic. When the patient can swallow easily, drinking lots of water should be encouraged.

DIABETES

Patients with diabetes who have control of their disease with daily monitoring of their blood sugar, insulin injections, and diet are capable of every outdoor activity. On cold trips, insulin should be carefully protected from freezing. Twice as much insulin, syringes, and batteries for the glucometer should be carried than would normally be needed, and these supplies should not all be carried by the same person.

A patient with diabetes may experience the dangerous rapid onset of *hypoglycemia* (low blood sugar), a *true emergency* characterized by an altered (confused) level of consciousness that often leads quickly to great hunger, pale skin, and unconsciousness. The patient should eat or drink something sugary as soon as possible. If she or he is unconscious, sugar or sugary substances, e.g., the commercial product Glutose, should be rubbed into the gums and under the tongue with the patient lying on his or her side. If hypoglycemia is untreated, death follows.

A patient with diabetes may also experience *hyper-glycemia* (high blood sugar) with accompanying great fatigue, great thirst, and the need to urinate. The onset of hyperglycemia is often slower than the onset of hypo-glycemia. Untreated high blood sugar leads to dehydration, a fruity odor on the breath, confusion, and coma. Treatment includes fluids and insulin. But insulin should *never* be injected except by a qualified physician. If unsure, give sugar—and evacuate the patient.

HEART ATTACK

Heart attack still leads to more deaths than any other cause in the United States. Patients complain of center-chest discomfort: crushing, squeezing pain or heavy pressure. Pain may radiate to the shoulder, down the arm, and into the jaw, predominantly on the left side. Nausea, sweating, and shortness of breath are common. Patients often deny the possibility that this could be a heart attack. In the backcountry there is little to be done other than 1) keeping the patient physically and emotional calm, in a position of comfort, and warm, and 2) giving one half an adult aspirin to reduce clotting of the blood. Do not allow the patient to walk. Help needs to be sought. If the patient has been prescribed nitroglycerin, one pill should be placed under the tongue with the patient sitting down. Most physicians recommend a second pill if the first fails to work, and a third if the second fails to work. *Consult your physician*.

HYPERVENTILATION SYNDROME

Far from home, pain and/or fear often cause the patient to breathe faster and deeper than normal. This hyperventilation may lead to chest tightness; tingling or numbness in the hands, feet, and/or face; and spasms in the hands and feet—which lead to more fear, which leads to more hyperventilation. The patient will either calm down or pass out. If he or she passes out, breathing may stop for what seems like a very long time. Except in rare circumstances the patient will indeed start breathing again. (*Note:* If he or she does not, give a few mouth-to-mouth breaths.) Hyperventilating patients need to be calmed and encouraged to breathe normally. When calmness returns, then you can investigate the cause of the pain or fear.

SEIZURES

A great variety of causes can produce the uncontrollable rigid, jerky muscular movements of a seizure (or convulsion). Many people suffer seizure disorders and take drugs to prevent seizures. During a seizure, which normally lasts no more than two minutes, the patient needs protection from harmful objects, but the patient does *not* need restraint. Do *not* place anything in the patient's mouth. After the seizure, the patient will usually feel extreme fatigue and the need to sleep. Let the patient rest, preferably in a side position to maintain an open airway. Do not leave the patient alone. Check for injuries that may have occurred during the seizure. The patient may require time and privacy to recover from some of the common results of a seizure, such as incontinence. Seizures for unknown reasons need a doctor's consultation. Seizures for known reasons should initiate heart-to-heart talks about the wisdom of continuing the trip.

UNCONSCIOUS STATES

An unconscious state is a condition in which the patient's level of consciousness has dropped below A (for Alert) on the AVPU scale (see "Patient Assessment System"). The patient cannot respond to your questions with answers you would very much like to have. An unconscious state is not always a medical emergency. Common causes in the backcountry include diabetic reactions, seizures, trauma, and alterations in normal body core temperature (all of which are addressed earlier in this book). To help you, hopefully, figure out why the patient has an altered mental status, ask what has caused the brain To STOP:

To: Toxins—poisons, with alcohol being a common causative factor

S: Sugar/Seizures—or, to put it in other words, diabetes and seizures

T: Temperature—alterations in normal body core temperature

O: Oxygen—in this case, the lack of it, as when an airway is blocked

P: Pressure—too much inside the head, often the result of brain swelling from injury

Principles for managing this patient include 1) stabilizing the spine (see "Spinal Injuries"); 2) maintaining an open airway, which may involve a side position for the patient; 3) searching thoroughly for "hidden" clues, e.g., on the ground nearby, in pockets, in a backpack, on medical alert tags; 4) considering giving sugar (see "Diabetes," above); and 5) monitoring the patient closely for changes in level of consciousness. Any patient with an altered mental status should be evacuated from the backcountry.

21. Gender-Specific Problems

FOR WOMEN ONLY

Alterations in normal menstrual cycles are not unusual for women in the outdoors. Unusual abdominal pain, however, associated with abnormal vaginal bleeding are indications for an evacuation. If there is a possibility of pregnancy associated with pain and vaginal bleeding, the patient should be *rapidly* evacuated. Pelvic pain with fever and chills, nausea and vomiting, and perhaps a watery, foul-smelling vaginal discharge also require a physician's attention.

More common and typically less serious symptoms of *vaginal infection* include excessive redness, itching, and perhaps an increase in vaginal discharge. Although there are several possible causes of such symptoms, treatment for any vaginitis may include washing the area thoroughly and air drying. Women with a history of vaginal infections should carry appropriate medications, such as Gyne-Lotrimin or Monistat or the prescription medication Diflucan. If treatment is not followed by improvement within forty-eight hours, an evacuation should be considered.

Urinary tract infections (UTI) cause increased frequency and urgency of urination, often with a burning sensation on urination. Fatigue and low abdominal pain are common. Blood or pus may appear in the urine. The patient should drink lots of water and avoid sugary foods and foods that irritate the bladder, e.g., caffeine, alcohol, and peppery foods. The perineal area should be washed daily with water and mild soap. On extended trips women should consider carrying an antibiotic for UTI. Ciprofloxacin (sold as Cipro) is often prescribed. *Consult your physician.* (*Note:* Men are not immune to UTI.) Evacuate any patient who does not respond to treatment, especially if the patient develops tenderness over the kidneys.

FOR MEN ONLY

Epididymitis, an inflammation of the epididymis, tends to come on slowly (but not always), possibly with a fever and a red, swollen, painful scrotum. The patient suffers, and the only immediate relief is found in rest, support for the scrotum (e.g., jockstrap or improvised support from a triangular bandage), painkillers, and cool compress to the affected area. Antibiotics are necessary. Evacuate the patient to a physician.

Torsion of the testis is a twisting of the testis within the scrotum. Pain may come on suddenly or slowly. Scrotum is red, swollen, and painful. The lack of blood supply means death for the testis in as quickly as a few hours. Evacuate the patient. Cool compresses and painkillers provide some relief. A jockstrap or improvised support may give some more relief and may increase blood flow to the testis. If the evacuation will be long, attempt to rotate the painful testis into a normal position. Since most testicles rotate inward, a gentle rotation outward may give immediate and blessed relief. The patient may wish to make the rotation himself. If this does not work, perhaps the testicle rotated in the opposite direction, so rotate the testicle two turns in the opposite direction. If you fail with these two attempts, the patient is no worse off than before the attempt was made.

22. Common Simple Problems

BLISTERS

Those fluid-filled bubbles are mild burns caused by friction. Friction produces a separation of the tough outer layer of skin from the sensitive inner layer. Only where skin is hardened is it thick enough for this to happen—heels, toes, soles, palms. Loose skin just wears away with friction, leaving an abrasion. Blisters range from unpleasant to terribly debilitating, but they are not a serious problem unless they become infected.

What should you do? Controlled draining is far better than having them rupture inside a dirty sock. Clean around the site thoroughly. Sterilize the point of a needle or knife and use it or a sterile scalpel to open the blister. Massage the fluid out. Leaving the roof of the blister intact will make it feel better and heal faster. If the roof has been rubbed away, treat

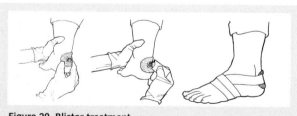

Figure 20. Blister treatment

the wound as you would any other (see "Wound and Wound Infection Management"). Apply a dressing that limits friction: Spenco 2nd Skin, or a moleskin "donut" (a rounded piece of moleskin with a hole cut in the center) filled with ointment, or ointment and a gauze pad over the blister. Whatever you put over the drained blister requires tape or moleskin strips to hold it in place.

Blisters can be prevented by 1) wearing boots or shoes that fit and are broken in; 2) wearing a thin inner sock under a thicker outer sock; 3) treating "hot spots" with moleskin, 2nd Skin, tape, or tincture of benzoin compound *before* they become blisters; and 4) taking off your boots to let your feet dry when you take a break from hiking.

DIARRHEA

The backcountry is home to a multitude of diarrhea-causing life-forms: protozoa, bacteria, viruses. Generally speaking, they will produce one of two kinds of diarrhea: 1) *Noninvasive diarrhea*, with microbial colonies on upper small intestine walls, leading to abdominal cramping, nausea, vomiting, and massive amounts of water, filled with salt and potassium, rushing out of the bowels. 2) *Invasive diarrhea*, sometimes called dysentery, with bacteria attacking the lower small intestine and colon, causes inflammation, bloody bowel movements, fever, abdominal cramping, and painful release of loose stools.

Whatever the cause, dehydration is the immediate problem with diarrhea. Mild diarrhea can be treated with water, diluted clear fruit juices, or sports drinks. Persistent diarrhea requires more aggressive replacement of electrolytes lost in the stool. Oral rehydration solutions are best for treating serious diarrhea. You can usually make do by adding one teaspoon of salt and eight teaspoons of sugar to a liter of water. The patient should drink about one-fourth of this solution every hour, along with all the water he or she will tolerate. Rice, grains, bananas, and potatoes are okay to eat. Fats, dairy products, caffeine, and alcohol should be avoided.

Over-the-counter medications for watery diarrhea, such as Imodium, are available and effective. Prescription medications include Lomotil. Dysentery should be treated with antibiotics. *Consult your physician concerning prescription drugs.* Patients with diarrhea lasting twenty-four to seventy-two hours should be evacuated (see "Abdominal Pain" in the "Medical Emergencies" section).

DEHYDRATION

Water is easily and quickly lost from the body in the outdoors through sweating, urination, breathing, and diarrhea. Even mild dehydration causes loss of energy, loss of mental acuity, and loss of fun. Mild dehydration shows up as thirst, dry mouth, and dark yellow urine. Moderate dehydration adds very dry mouth, reduction of the amount of dark urine, a rapid weak pulse, and remarkable dizziness when the patient stands up. Severe dehydration causes very, very dry mouth, lack of urine, and shock. Treatment of dehydration is explained above (see "Diarrhea"). Prevention is this: Drink lots of clear fluids, especially water. Drink a half-liter every morning. Drink regularly and often during periods of exercise. Drink enough to keep your urine clear.

DENTAL PROBLEMS

Where a filling has fallen out or a cavity has developed, pain usually first occurs when cold, food, or your tongue hits the spot. After rinsing the area clean, a drop of oil of cloves (eugenol) will ease the pain. A temporary filling is the best treatment until a dentist can be found. Cavit is the easiest to use and best temporary filling material. Just fill the hole with Cavit, bite to align with the teeth above, and wait till it hardens. A temporary filling can be made by mixing zinc oxide powder and eugenol. To improvise, fill the cavity with candle wax, ski wax, or sugarless gum. Temporary filling material can also be used to hold a dislodged crown back in place.

If a tooth is knocked out, there is a small chance it can be salvaged if you can get it back in the hole from whence it came. After rinsing the tooth off (do *not* scrub it), press it gently back in place. If it will not go back in, at least hold on to it until you find a dentist. Same goes for a piece of tooth that has broken off.

When a broken tooth exposes the pulp, pain can be extreme. A small piece of aspirin placed directly on the exposed pulp causes a burning pain but "cauterizes" the pulp, putting an end to the patient's distress for a while. *Never* put aspirin on the gum next to an aching tooth. Acid in aspirin will burn the gum. Swallow the aspirin, or another painkiller, if you need further relief.

Any bleeding inside the mouth can be given direct pressure with a gauze pad held in place with your finger or bitten in place with your teeth. A moistened nonherbal tea bag can be used instead of gauze. Avoid irritating a wound in the mouth: no smoking, no chewing on the "bad" side, no hot foods, no sucking on the wound.

An infected tooth is indicated by a lot of swelling in the gum and cheek near the tooth. Discoloration may be visible. This tooth needs a dentist as soon as possible. Cold packs on the cheek may give some relief. If evacuation is delayed, have the patient rinse her or his mouth several times a day with warm, salty water. It would be best to start the patient on an oral antibiotic. *Consult your physician* concerning antibiotics for tooth infection.

And consult your dentist at least one month prior to an extended backcountry trip or a journey to a foreign country to have potential problems identified and treated. Routine oral hygiene will prevent most trip-ruining dental problems: Floss once a day and brush twice a day with a soft-bristled toothbrush.

EAR PROBLEMS

Do not poke anything in your ear smaller than your elbow. If something is lodged in the ear, such as a small insect, try flushing it out with alcohol or water. Outer ear infections, or "swimmer's ear," hurt more when you pull on the earlobe. Flush the ear daily with dilute vinegar or alcohol. If pain persists, find a doctor. Middle ear infections do not increase in pain when the earlobe is tugged and are often accompanied by vertigo. These infections require antibiotic treatment—see a doctor.

EYE PROBLEMS

If the patient complains of something in the eye, look closely and try to identify the object. If it is lodged, leave it alone and find a doctor. If it is large and lodged, protect the object to prevent it being bumped, and carry out the patient sitting at approximately a 45 degree angle. If it is small and loose, flush it out or dab it out with a soft cloth. Once loose objects are removed, the patient may complain that it still feels like something is there. The eye is probably scratched—typically not serious, but the eye will heal faster patched shut for twenty-four hours. A black eye is typically not serious and self-limiting, but beware of injuries that produce visible cuts or any disturbance in vision—reasons to find a doctor. Swollen, red, itchy eyes with a colorful discharge are almost always infected. After flushing the eye with disinfected water, small amounts of antibiotic ointment may be placed in the eye several times a day. Ointments made for the eye are best. If the problem persists, it should be seen by a physician.

FISHHOOK REMOVAL

The *string-pull technique* requires a loop of string: Place the loop around the curve of the hook, push down on the hook to loosen the barb, yank the loop—the hook pops out. The *push-through-and-snip technique* requires pushing the embedded hook out through the skin, snipping off the barb, and backing the hook out. If it is a large and deeply embedded hook, you will have to slice delicately with a sharp edge to loosen the hook prior to removal.

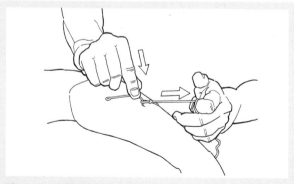

Figure 21. Fishhook removal

HEADACHE

A common outdoor complaint, headaches have three general causes: 1) dehydration, 2) muscular tension, and 3) a vascular disorder. Most headaches respond to rest, hydration, massage, and over-the-counter painkillers, e.g., ibuprofen. Beware of the headache that comes on suddenly, is unrelieved by rest and medication, and is not like any other headache you have ever had—reasons to find a doctor.

NOSEBLEED

Lean the patient forward and pinch the meaty part of the nose firmly shut. Hold it for ten to fifteen minutes. If bleeding persists, a squirt of a nose spray, such as Afrin, may help stop the bleeding. If the bleeding still persists, pack the nostrils gently with gauze soaked with antibiotic ointment or a spray such as Afrin. Most nosebleeds are not serious, but it is possible for noses to bleed from the back so that blood runs down the throat. These posterior nosebleeds need a physician's attention.

SNOWBLINDNESS

Six to twelve hours after overexposure to the sun's radiation, the patient complains of pain and swelling in the eye with a feeling like an "eye full of sand." The cornea of the eye has been sunburned. Sunburned eyes are usually very sensitive to light. Rinses with cool water will clean the eye and ease the pain. Cool compresses may be applied for pain. A small amount of antibiotic ointment may be applied several times a day for two to three days. Ointments made for the eye are best. The patient's eyes may need to be covered for twenty-four hours. Snowblindness almost always resolves harmlessly in twenty-four to forty-eight hours. Prolonged discomfort is reason to see a physician. The problem can be prevented by wearing sunglasses that block UV radiation. On snow or water, sunglasses should fit well and have side shields to block reflected UV light.

SPLINTERS

Splinters should be removed as soon as possible. If the end is visible, grasp it with tweezers and pull it out gently. If the end is buried, probe with your fingers until you find the orientation of the splinter, and push it toward the wound until the end is graspable. In the case of deeply buried splinters, you may need to cut superficially with a sterile scalpel to expose the embedded object. Clean and dress any resulting wounds.

SUNBURN

The immediate response to overexposure to ultraviolet light is burned skin. Prolonged exposure, over years, leads to premature skin aging and degenerative skin disorders such as cancer. First aid for sunburn includes cooling the skin, applying a moisturizer, taking ibuprofen for pain and inflammation, and staying out of direct sunlight. If blisters form, a doctor should be consulted. Prevention of sunburn includes wearing hats with brims and tightly woven clothing, sunblocks such as zinc oxide, and sunscreens with a high sun protection factor—SPF 15 or more. Be aware: You can burn on cloudy days, sunlight is most harmful between the hours of 10:00 A.M. and 3:00 P.M., and large amounts of UV light are reflected by snow and water.

WATER DISINFECTION

A lot of gastrointestinal distress can be avoided at home and abroad if you disinfect all drinking water. There are three methods that work:

1. **Boiling** will kill organisms that make people sick. In fact, the time it takes water to reach the boiling point, even at high altitudes, kills organisms. So by the time water has reached the point of boiling, it is safe to drink.

2. **Filters** differ greatly in their ability to disinfect water. Some filter out only protozoa, such as Giardia and Cryptosporidium. Some filter out protozoa and bacteria. None filter out viruses, but some have an iodine-resin on the filter that may kill viruses. Choose carefully.

3. **Chemicals** can be added to water to kill harmful organisms. Products containing iodine or chlorine are generally the safest and most effective, but few chemicals guarantee

water safe from Cryptosporidium (with Potable Aqua chlorine dioxide tablets being one exception). Iodine is commercially available in several forms including Potable Aqua iodine tablets and iodine crystals. If you have povidone-iodine solution in your first-aid kit, it can be used to disinfect water. The solution is best measured with a dropper. Eight drops of povidone-iodine solution in a liter of warm, clear water and a fifteen-minute wait will give you a safe drink. For cold, clear water, double the drops and double the wait (sixteen drops for thirty minutes). For cloudy water, double the drops and triple the wait.

23. First Aid for Children

When traveling into remote geographical locations with children, your medical knowledge and your first-aid kit should be adapted to meet their special smaller bodies. Although specific needs may differ from trip to trip depending on such variables as the ages of the children, the length of the trip, the time of year of the trip, and any preexisting medical conditions, some medical advice is useful for all younger ages.

KIDS AND HEAT

Children gain core heat faster than adults. Little human cooling systems work fine, most of the time, but they sometimes need encouragement. The younger the child the less developed his or her internal heat regulating system, and the larger the surface area for heat dissipation in relation to body mass.

Allow your children time to acclimatize to heat. It will take them longer than it will take you. Early in the hot season or early into a trip to an area hotter than your child is used to, go easy for the first few days. Increase the activity level progressively. The human body becomes increasingly able to withstand the heat.

Encourage your children to drink lots of water. And do not be surprised if they claim a lack of thirst. Children feel the need to drink less readily than adults. Thirst is often a sign that the body has already entered the early stages of dehydration. The old proverb advising "you can't drink too much water" is technically false but practically true. Water loss from your child can be significant during one hour of activity in a warm climate. If you find it difficult to get kids to drink plain water, add enough powdered flavoring to make the water less boring, but not enough to make it syrupy.

KIDS AND DIARRHEA

Children dehydrate faster than adults, and fluid loss, especially via diarrhea, can be devastating. One of the best and earliest signs of dehydration is urine color: Clear indicates a well-hydrated child (or adult) and dark yellow indicates poor hydration. As dehydration grows worse, watch for headache, unusual fatigue, loss of appetite, nausea, and other complaints that make you think flu. One of the later signs of serious dehydration in a child is restlessness and unusual loss of interest in whatever is going on around him or her.

For treating diarrhea, carry a mild antidiarrheal medication in your first aid kit. Children should continue to eat during episodes of diarrhea. Avoid milk for a day. Infants do well on rice cereal, applesauce, and bananas for a day or two. Older children may eat plain dry toast, plain crackers, plain chicken soup, and other bland foods. After the first couple of days, eating yogurt helps to repopulate the bowels with healthy bacteria.

KIDS AND DEHYDRATION

For treating dehydration, whether from diarrhea, vomiting, or heat, use oral rehydration salts (ORS) instead of plain water. ORS replace essential salts and contain a little sugar for energy. You can buy ORS or make your own rehydration solution by adding eight teaspoons of sugar and a teaspoon of salt to one liter of water. Do *not* use salt tablets.

KIDS AND SUNSHINE

The sun is worse on kids than it is on adults, even though the damage may not show up for thirty years. Eighty percent of skin damage from the sun (including skin cancers) happens in the first couple of decades of life.

Children sunburn more easily than adults. Children should wear clothing woven tightly enough to protect their skin from ultraviolet light, hats with a brim to protect their faces, and sunscreen on unprotected skin. Ultraviolet A and B damage skin, and the sunscreen should protect against both. Assume the sun protection factor (SPF) is not as strong as it claims and use a higher number. Sunscreens should be applied in a uniform coat over all exposed areas. If your trip involves swimming, use a waterproof sunscreen, and reapply it often. A few inches of water will not protect your child's skin from sunburn. Once a pleasant suntan is established, the screen should still be used. Tans prevent burning but offer little protection from the harmful effects of the sun.

Keep children under one year out of the sun as much as possible, and apply sunscreens to their sensitive skin only when absolutely necessary. Test the screen on a small portion of skin, about the size of your hand, first to see if the child will react. If she or he does react, try a different brand. For young children use a screen prepared as a milky lotion or cream, and avoid applying it to the upper and lower eyelids, where the screen might be rubbed involuntarily into the eye. Never use baby oil in the sun. Encourage children to wear sunglasses to reduce the chance of cataracts later in life and to protect their sensitive eyelids.

If your child gets sunburned, start treatment as soon as possible. Cool compresses may reduce the pain and limit the depth of the burn. Moisturizing lotions should be applied to skin. Acetaminophen may be given for pain. Drinking lots of water is important in the treatment of sunburn.

KIDS AND INSECTS

Children usually have more trouble than adults resisting the temptation to scratch itchy bites. Because youngsters are also typically less hygienic than adults, scratches on children have a higher rate of infection. Sting wipes may be used immediately to reduce the temptation to scratch. Hydrocortisone cream will reduce the itch of more established bites. To improvise an anti-itch medication, you may use a slurry of baking soda or meat tenderizer. Bites that are scratched open should be washed with soap and water and covered with an adhesive strip dressing.

For prevention, insect repellent should be used regularly. Deet, a common repelling ingredient, should not be used in a high concentration. For children the lower the concentration the better. Keep the repellent off childrens' hands and you will reduce the chance they will rub it into their eyes or, worse, suck it off their fingers. You can avoid deet by choosing products made with natural repellents, such as lemon eucalyptus oil (which has been proven as effective as approximately an 8 percent concentration of deet).

KIDS AND POISONS

Campsites should be checked closely to identify the pres-
ence of poison oak, sumac, or ivy. Children should be made
aware of, and taught how to identify and avoid, all poisonous
plants. If contact is suspected, all skin that may have contacted the poisonous plant should be washed immediately
with soft soap and cool water. Clothing, including shoes,
which may have contacted the poisonous plant should be
cleaned thoroughly. If the itch, redness, and fluid-filled bumps
of a reaction to the plants develop on skin, hydrocortisone
cream or calamine lotion may be used to treat the symptoms. Only time will bring healing.

Small children make up the majority of ingested-poison
patients. In the case of a suspected poisoning, consider
inducing vomiting as soon as possible. The child should first
be given water to drink—at least eight ounces. Then gently
stimulate the gag reflex with your finger. Do not induce vomiting in children who 1) are having seizures, 2) are lethargic or
in danger of further loss of consciousness, 3) have already
vomited, 4) have ingested a corrosive substance (which usually produces burns on the lips or in the mouth), or 5) have
ingested a petroleum product. If the child has ingested a poison, he or she should be evacuated to a medical facility as
soon as possible, even if vomiting has occurred. Prevent poisoning by clearly identifying to the child anything in the envi-

ronment that should be avoided, and keeping all dangerous substances out of reach.

KIDS AND MEDICATIONS

Children aged five and under usually cannot swallow pills. Carry chewable tablets. For children too little to chew, the tablets can be crushed and added to food. Some children's medications are available in liquid form, less desirable for backcountry trips, but it might be your best choice. For pain and/or fever, acetaminophen and/or ibuprofen are typically recommended. You may wish to carry an antihistamine. Consult your physician.

KIDS GET LOST

To help prevent children from wandering off indiscreetly into the wild places, set strict boundaries around campsites. Supply children with whistles and a code: Three blows means "Help!" . . . two blows means "We hear you!" Encourage children to hug a tree (stay put) if they get lost.

KIDS AND OUCHIES

Little people get scraped and cut and blistered just like big people (see "Wound and Wound Infection Management"), but they sometimes make less-than-perfect patients. To encourage cooperation carry kid-oriented wound management products, e.g., adhesive strips with cartoon characters on them.

24. Advice to International Travelers

Do not leave the United States (or get out of bed) without first understanding the risks you may be taking and how to prepare for them.

VACCINATIONS

Check with your physician and the Centers for Disease Control (CDC) about what vaccinations to get and other precautions to take before entering the foreign countries on your itinerary. Allow six to eight weeks to make sure you have time to get everything done that they recommend.

Current recommendations for U.S. travelers issued by the CDC are found in *Health Information for International Travel* (published annually). This publication contains vaccination and certification requirements on a country-by-country basis. It has the U.S. Public Health Service recommendations for difficult immunization questions—such as immunization of infants and breast-feeding or pregnant women—and specific recommendations for vaccination and prophylaxis for each of a wide variety of disorders. It also contains a discussion of specific potential health hazards worldwide by geographic region. The information in this book is updated in the biweekly *Summary of Health Information for International Travel*. Both the book and updates can be obtained from the Superintendent of Documents, U.S. Government Printing Office, Washington, DC 20402. They are also carried by many major libraries, nearly all health departments, and travelers' clinics.

In general all travelers should make sure their childhood immunizations are up to date, immunizations that include polio, measles, mumps, diphtheria, and whooping cough. All travelers should be assured of their tetanus immunity and should consider acquiring immunity to hepatitis A and B.

MALARIA

Malaria ranks as a leading cause of death on this planet. Once thought to result from breathing "swamp gas," the moist fumes rising from wet areas, *malaria* literally means "bad air." But all four species of the parasite that cause the disease get into human blood only from the bite of the female *Anopheles* mosquito. Malaria is the greatest disease risk to U.S. travelers to any region where the disease exists.

Your ounce of prevention should include everything possible to avoid mosquito bites (see "Bites and Stings"). These precautions, unfortunately, seldom meet all your prevention needs, and accidental exposure to an infected mosquito is virtually guaranteed in high-risk areas.

So to be as safe as possible, you will have to resort to chemical prophylaxis. The drug of choice for prevention of malaria has long been chloroquine (and it still is in some regions of the world), but some parasites have developed a resistance to it. In March 1990 the CDC made mefloquine the officially approved drug in chloroquine-resistant areas. Some people, however, experience side effects with mefloquine. Malarone is a newer and more expensive drug being recommended by a growing number of doctors. In all cases, *consult your physician*.

FOOD AND WATER

Amoebic dysentery, diarrheal diseases, and parasitic worms are associated with poor choice of water and food in many countries. Disinfect all water before drinking, brushing your teeth, or mixing your cocktails. Avoid milk, butter, and other dairy products. Watch bottled drinks being uncapped before you accept one. Make sure all food is well cooked and served hot. Fruits with intact skins are safe if peeled shortly before consumption. Do not go swimming in backcountry lakes, ponds, and streams where there is any chance of acquiring the fluke that causes schistosomiasis.

SOURCES OF INFORMATION

Questions about special health considerations and new developments in things to watch out for will be answered on the CDC's 24-hour automated International Traveler's Hotline: (877) FYI–TRIP. Or go to www.cdc.gov.

You might also consider packing the International Association for Medical Assistance to Travelers (IAMAT) list of worldwide English-speaking physicians. The list is free of charge: IAMAT, 417 Center Street, Lewiston, NY 14092; (716) 754–4883.

An alternative source of information is the publication *International Travel and Health,* published yearly by the World Health Organization (WHO). You can download this publication at www.who.int/ith/en, but it is less comprehensive than the CDC publication.

MEDICAL KITS

All international travelers should carry their own first-aid kit, especially trekkers who end up well away from medical assistance of any sort. Kits designed by professionals are available from several manufacturers, including Atwater Carey. Your physician will probably be willing to help you add the hard-to-find items you may want to have along. The kit should include a brief written personal medical history including allergies and recent illnesses, and any prescription drugs you are personally using with written directions for their use and—in case you remind some border guard of a smuggler—a copy of the prescription. *Note:* If you use or think you will need an injected drug, carry your own sterile syringes. It is not safe to rely on the sterility of needles in many countries. Carry painkillers, antacids, antihistamines, antidiarrhea medications, insect repellent, sunscreen, a means to disinfect water, a few basic splinting materials, and wound management materials including ointment, gauze, and tape and other bandages. Check your kit before every trip to make sure 1) you have what you might need, and 2) everything is up to date, particularly medications. Remember a first-aid kit functions only at the level of the person using it. If you really want to take care of yourself and others in remote settings, pack some training into your brain.

About the Author

Buck Tilton, MS, WEMT, has more than thirty years of experience in first aid and extended care. Known and respected worldwide, he has spent most of his adult life instructing outdoor enthusiasts in wilderness medicine. He is cofounder of the Wilderness Medicine Institute of the National Outdoor Leadership School in Lander, Wyoming. He has written more than 1,000 magazine articles and authored or coauthored twenty-four books, including *Wilderness First Responder, Medicine for the Backcountry*, and *Basic Essentials of Rescue in the Backcountry.* In addition to his many writing and teaching responsibilities, Tilton serves as a medical consultant to Wisconsin Pharmacal Company in Jackson, Wisconsin. He lives in Lander with his wife, Kat, his son, Zachary, and his daughter, BaoXin Cheyenne.